adventures in sex

adventures in
sex

365 ways to make every day & night more exciting

MARK BRICKLIN

Founding editor, *Men's Health* magazine

Stewart, Tabori & Chang
New York

Published in 2005 by
Stewart, Tabori & Chang
115 West 18th Street
New York, NY 10011
www.abramsbooks.com

Library of Congress Cataloging-in-Publication Data
Bricklin, Mark.
    Adventures in sex : 365 ways to make every night & day more exciting /
    By Mark Bricklin.
    p. cm.
  ISBN: 1-58479-461-5
    1. Sex instruction. 2. Sex. 3. Sexual excitement. I. Title.
HQ31.B7795 2005
613.9'6—dc22   2005016412

Designed by Galen Smith & Allyson McFarlane
The text of this book was composed in Trade Gothic and Chalet.

Printed in the United States of America

10 9 8 7 6 5 4 3 2 1

First Printing

Stewart, Tabori & Chang is a subsidiary of

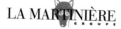

LA MARTINIÈRE

To my loving and brilliant wife, Lynn, who helped me in the writing of this book in more ways than I can ever say.

Most authors of sex books approach their subject as if it were a sport, like naked golf, or perhaps a craft, like extremely naughty needlepoint. And that's fine, as far as it goes.

But sex is more than a sport. It's more than a craft. It's more than any one thing. Sex is an entire dimension of life, along with intellect, emotion, memory, body chemistry, even spirituality. And sex not only rubs shoulders with these other dimensions, it dances with them. They change how sex is experienced, and sex changes them. Yes: though few people realize it, sex affects our total sense of life happiness, our body chemistry (right down to the molecular level!), and, believe it or not, extends our life expectancy.

Because so many things not usually considered part of "sex" actually improve or harm it, this book is more wide-ranging than other sex books. It will tell you things you never heard before, and things you won't believe even though I swear they're true!

Adventures in Sex will tell you, for example:

- Why the pleasure centers of you brain are programmed to go into seventh heaven when you and your lover perform certain sex acts, like Reverse Oral Sex, The Escalator of Love, or Conquering Hero Sex.
- How to teach your man what turns you on, and what gets you off, without seeming like a naked schoolmarm.
- How to teach your woman to play your penis like a French horn, a trombone—a whole orchestra!
- The breakfast food that boosts the hormone of desire with every spoonful.

- Devices you never dreamed existed...that will give you sexual sensations you never dreamed existed!
- Exercises scientifically proven to increase your sexual desire and performance by leaps and bounds!
- How to bring your wildest sexual fantasies to vibrant *I-can't-believe-I'm-finally-doing-this!* life. (Though not necessarily on the first date!)
- Delightful aromas you can create at home, medically proven to get your juices flowing—literally!
- Devious little tricks to do at the last minute to turn a good orgasm into a screamer.
- How to turn a chronic grump into a sweeter, more loving person with this certain food. A miracle? Medical research says it really works!
- Intimate, sexy outfits so "secret" they don't sell them even at Victoria's Secret!
- The astonishing but best way to put a woman in the mood for sex. A totally different best way to get a guy in the mood.
- How to increase the natural body compound that should be called the real Love Potion No.9.
- Foods that stiffen a man's erection. Foods that stifle it. Foods scientifically proven to make a woman more hungry for sex, and her sensations stronger and sweeter.

In short, *Adventures in Sex* will give you hundreds of bed-tested ways to reach higher levels of sexual rapture than ever before. Knock yourself out! **—M.B.**

January

pleasure and
surprise

1 NEW YEAR'S DAY

This year will be more exciting and pleasurable for you and your lover even if you are well on the way to knowing each other's favorite bedtime frolics. And that, largely thanks to a scientific technology that didn't even exist a few years ago!

The discovery: *When you are stimulated in a way you did not expect to be, the pleasure centers of your brain do back flips.*

Maybe science is just catching up with what you already knew by experience. In any case, research done with special MRI equipment at Emory University and Baylor College of Medicine was able to track changes in the activity of a known brain pleasure center (called the nucleus accumbens) as different patterns of stimulation were given to participants. The doctors expected that as people got heavy doses of what they liked most, their brains would light up like a jukebox. Only they didn't.

"We found the reward pathways responded much more strongly to the unexpectedness of stimuli instead of their pleasurable effects," the researchers reported. "This means the brain finds unexpected pleasures more rewarding than expected ones, and"—this is my favorite part—"it may have little to do with what people say they like."

Other researchers have found that novel experiences drive up levels of both testosterone and dopamine, two key ingredients in the recipe for hot sex. Further, according to Helen Fisher, Ph.D., it's been shown in lab experiments that when people share novel, exciting experiences, it increases the attraction they feel toward one another.

MORAL: **Keep an open mind as you read on.**

provocative fact #1
are you
well-educated?

Researchers at the University of Chicago have found that, compared to women who never finished high school, women who attended college are twice as likely to give or receive oral sex.

"breastercourse"
technique #1
man on top

3 There's scarcely a word in most sex manuals about a man thrusting his penis between his partner's breasts, while she's pushing them together. Probably it strikes these authors that this kind sex is somehow lewd... crude... even rude, especially if the man shoots his wad on the woman's chin. That's why I'm including it. Lewd is good. Lewd, crude, and rude can be even better.

The woman does not have to have especially large breasts to perform what I call "breastercourse" (there's another term for it, but it's...lewd). So long as she can hold her breasts together in such a way that the man can move his penis up and down, it will work fine.

A lubricant is highly recommended for breastercourse. Be sure to use one that either has no smell at all, or a pleasant flowery aroma she likes, because the stuff is going to be pretty close to her nose.

The man must be careful to support nearly all of his weight on his knees and shins, or he will squash the woman. The woman may want a pillow under her head to feel more comfortable, or to get a better view of the action.

This maneuver can be carried through to climax (and it may take some time) or can be used as an intermission between other approaches. If used as the climactic act, the man, after checking with his partner, can either aim his penis toward the pillow when he comes, or fire dead ahead for a special treat—for him, anyway!

---

swiss **balling**

4 Nearly every gym you visit today has Swiss balls—big, beach ball–type globes that people drape themselves over to do various exercises. I've seen them employed for all sorts of exercises: crunches, leg lifts, push-ups, rowing with dumbbells, you name it. They add an extra dimension of difficulty that makes each exercise that much more beneficial (i.e., harder).

If you have a Swiss ball in your home gym, you can also use it to have sex—with a degree of difficulty added. The woman can sprawl on top of the ball with her legs spread. The man places his legs outside of hers, then enters her. In all likelihood, the ball is going to start rolling. That's where the difficulty—and fun—comes in.

She can also lie on the ball tummy-down. Vaginal entrance might be tricky at this angle but anal entrance is easier. Again, prepare for a little "trip around the world." Should one or both of you slide off, or simply break up laughing, so much the better. Laughing is one of the most underrated aphrodisiacs.

> SPECIAL NOTE: **Small Swiss balls are now available on sex toy websites.**

put more hootchy
in your kootchy

5 Sex involves a lot of hip and abdominal action, in case you haven't noticed. Here's a simple exercise that will give you greater strength and staying power, with the nice bonus of being great for your abs.

It's called the reverse crunch, because instead of lifting your torso toward your feet, you lift your legs over your torso. Lie on your back on the floor on a rug or mat, and bend your knees. *They will stay bent throughout the exercise.* Now lift your legs toward your head just far enough so that your butt is off the floor. Your feet do not have to actually go so far as to be directly over your head.

Do as many as you can in just one set and you're done. Repeat every other day, and you'll be able to do more and more. You... a sexual athlete!

---

paying homage to her
one-of-a-kind

The clitoris, say medical experts, is the only organ in the human body that has no other function than creating and transmitting pleasure. There are many ways to honor its singularity: One is written communication, specifically, the man using his tongue to spell messages on his partner's pleasure button. Make up your own message: "You're so hot!" is a good beginning. Don't tell her the message; let her be the decoder. It's easier, by the way, to spell out words in big capital letters, but those of adept and well-practiced tongue may provide additional exquisite pleasure by writing in cursive.

the missionary
position **for atheists**

7

If it were *that* bad, it wouldn't be the most common copulatory posture in the known universe, for one thing. Knocking it is like knocking McDonald's when you know damn well you'll be going there soon enough to fill your French fry hole.

It's also a good position for continuing the human race, it turns out. With the woman on her back, her vagina acts like a funnel, collecting sperm with the aid of gravity. And if her legs are stretched straight up and out, or rest on the man's shoulders as they "missionary," that makes for deeper penetration of sperm as well. One might speculate that at various times in history, when there were severe threats to human survival due to hard times, the missionary position might have even aided in the survival of our species.

Having said that, let's admit that for the woman, it's a little—or a lot—like being pinned for the count—a *long* count—in a wrestling match, while the man may find that he's climaxing too soon. Just as bad, the fact that you've made love this way 500 times before could create the feeling that you're having *rerun* sex.

There are a number of good variations on the standard "mish-posish" included in this book, and here's one for starters. Place a well-stuffed pillow under Madame's tush. The increased angle of entry should increase pleasure for both of you. With her hips elevated, she may find it nice to sort of drape her legs around the man's midsection. If his waist isn't too big, she can even play footsie with herself.

when to keep
your mouth closed

8

"Often the difference between a successful marriage and a mediocre one consists of leaving about three or four things a day unsaid." — Harlan Miller

The same goes for a successful sexual relationship. Despite our hormones, it's amazing how fast the desire to have sex can evaporate when we hear our partner say the wrong thing. Only rarely are they insults: Most often they are simply thoughtless comments that are demeaning. The speaker may not think what he or she said was a big deal; but to the receiving party, it hurts like a paper cut—pain completely out of proportion with a seemingly minor event.

My personal policy is never to say *anything* of a negative nature, even in jest. About her, her family, her household business management, anything whatsoever. Now, this policy is not meant to keep mum if your partner seems to be turning into a drug addict or has mysterious sores or if flames start shooting out of the toaster as we speak. It's about the things that really don't matter, even if they piss you off a little at the time. Three or four things a day: That's just about right. It'll do wonders for your sex life *and* your marriage!

Flying **Foreplay**

9

Where is it written that foreplay has to be done immediately prior to sex?

In every sex manual, you say?

I beg to differ. Foreplay can be profitably engaged in hours before actual sex. It creates a smoldering itch that *knows* it's going to get scratched, but doesn't know when.

You're both on a longish airplane ride, headed for vacation. Looking forward to good times, you begin to get horny. There're two minor problems. One, you want to save your best for when you arrive at your romantic vacation site. Second, you're on an airplane, and despite what you've heard about the "Mile High Club," the idea of doing it in the bathroom has no appeal whatsoever. Solution: flying foreplay.

She covers both of them with blankets and then subtly begins groping him. Maybe she even unzips him and touches him; not rubbing but just sort of holding him. A good time to do this is when there are food and drink carts in the aisle and no one is moving about the cabin. If they show a movie, that's the best time.

This is just teasing, remember. If you sense it's going too far, either stop at once or make sure you have napkins under the blankets.

Of course you don't have to be in an airplane to have "premature" foreplay. You could enjoy it at home... at the beach... dallying in the hot tub; wherever you have at least *some* bit of privacy. It will pay dividends later. You may even find that at least one partner will need no further foreplay; they're *ready*.

---

do it **with a duvet**

10

As the weather turns colder, or at least a little chillier if you live in the South, consider the exquisite pleasure of having sex under a duvet, instead of a bunch of sheets, blankets, spreads, quilts, and your Old English sheepdog. The freedom you have under a light, fluffy (but incredibly warm) duvet will amaze you if you haven't experienced one before. Plus, they have washable coverings so you don't have to worry about stains.

Best of all, even the neatest woman doesn't try to tuck in a duvet, so you don't get a hernia trying to roll over.

butter her **up**

11

"When he takes his sexual organ in his hand and rotates it in all directions [in his partner], it is called 'churning.'" So saith the love classic *Kama Sutra*, from ancient India, a land that even today is known for *ghee*, or clarified butter. Churn first around the opening and slowly work down. A slow, methodical tempo and "Tell me when it feels good" will both facilitate the buttering-up process.

turn back your **clitoral clock**

12

There is a device that, in effect, helps turn back the clock of aging for the clitoris, and other parts of the vagina as well. It can even help women who haven't yet bought their first pair of drugstore reading glasses.

It's called the Eros-CTD, the letters standing for clitoral therapy device. Designed to fit over the clitoris and surrounding area like an electronic tiara, the device produces a gentle sucking action (which the woman controls), which in turn enhances localized blood flow and sense of arousal.

This is not some sex toy, but a genuine medical sex aid that has been approved by the Food and Drug Administration. Prescribed by many physicians to women who need it, the Eros-CTD may do more than get a woman ready to enjoy sex on a given day or night. The theory, according to Doctors Jennifer and Laura Berman, "is that, over time, this will prevent fibrosis of the clitoris and labial arteries that occurs with age."

FOR MORE INFORMATION: **UroMetrics.com.**

if food be the music of love, **chew on**

13 Folklore is replete with notions of foods that make you sexier—oysters, most notably—but their effect comes mostly (or entirely) from suggestion. While suggestion can be pretty powerful stuff, there's something even more powerful. Mary Polan, M.D., asserts unequivocally that L-arginine, an amino acid, "is the only nutrient that has been proved to increase sexual arousal in women." L-arginine is found abundantly in peanuts (and peanut butter), but goobers are not the world's most romantic food. Luckily, another excellent source of the naughty nutrient is walnuts, which are far higher up the scale of culinary sophistication.

Here's a 5-star yet easy walnut recipe from Sara Moulton, of the TV show *Cooking Live*, that you can enjoy as a snack, appetizer, or dessert.

ROSEMARY WALNUTS

2½ tablespoons unsalted butter
2 teaspoons crumbled dried rosemary
1 teaspoon salt
½ teaspoon cayenne pepper
2 cups walnut halves

Simply melt the butter with seasonings in a small saucepan. Place the walnuts in a medium bowl and pour the butter over them. Toss to coat, then bake on a cookie sheet in a preheated 350°F oven for 10 minutes.

"welcome to my vagina"

14

This is a polite, considerate, and pleasing way for a man to open a woman with his hands. He begins by placing either the heel of his palm, or the inside of his knuckle bones on the woman's pubic mound, the soft area of flesh with the pubic hair. Which part of the hand is placed there will depend of the size of the man's hand and on the size of the woman. In any case, the man's fingers should be able to cup just about all of her outer vagina when his hand is duly in place.

He cups her for a moment as a gesture of affection, then he gets his pinkie out of the picture so that his three fingers are over her. Slowly he begins tracing between her outer lips with his middle finger. *Slowly.* The idea here is to let her response dictate her opening (and that's *not* a pun), as much as the persuasion of his eager digits. His surrounding fingers can gently help along the sides.

When she opens sufficiently, he adds more gentle persuasion by placing his other hand on top of the busy hand. Rather than make only parallel movements, hand number two can also sneak in for some complementary moves, such as little circles over her clitoris.

Then he moves one hand down to the bottom of her vagina and inserts a finger in a few inches, curling the tip along the side to stimulate her G-spot. Meanwhile, his other hand is still entertaining her clitoris.

Important: Ask her if you're doing it the way she likes it. Because tonight she may feel different than she did last night. This is a reliable warmer-upper, but can also be continued or expanded upon (orally, for instance, or with a vibrator) to bring her to climax.

---

talk with your eyes

15 Communicating, or just plain talking, to use an old-fashioned word, is one of the most important enhancers of good sex. It's better even than champagne. But what if one person in the conversation is an oral no-show? He (90 percent of the time it *is* a he) seems tongue-tied, and you're getting pretty frustrated.

Use this technique, which actually underwent R&D by specialists in social interaction (yet another fancy term for talking).

Look at him with steady eye contact the whole time you're speaking. But when you're done, and you want *him* to chime in, *look away*, a mere second or two later. If you stare at him, he will feel like you're pressuring him, like a detective on *Law and Order* interrogating a suspect. Turn the spotlight off and let him take a breath.

the hidden appeal of
the missionary
position

16 Besides its familiarity and general utilitarian nature, there is a hidden appeal to the missionary position few of us have ever imagined. With the man on top and the woman literally pinned down, what you have is the pirate-grapples-with-fair-maiden effect. Or, in the words of Jude Carter, Ph.D., a shrink and sex therapist, "Sometimes a man likes to dominate a woman; there are some times when a woman likes to be 'taken' by a man." With any luck, these "sometimes" will occur at the same time for both partners.

TIP TO MEN: Holding her wrists down above her head increases your Morgan the Pirate persona.

TIP TO WOMEN: Squirming as if you can't decide whether you want to escape his brutal grip or pleasure yourself against his salty loins will make you a wetter wench and Morgan a happy pirate.

this is your brain.
this is your brain on orgasm.

17

Men are notorious for going into a kind of stupor after climaxing, a stupor that too often leads to unconsciousness (also known as sleep). His partner may think he's inconsiderate, selfish, not willing to provide some good afterglow...or even help her to the climax she hasn't yet enjoyed.

Before you condemn your man, though, listen to this. Using the brain-scanning technique of functional MRI, scientists have discovered that when a man climaxes, his entire frontal cortex (the part of the brain that does most of the thinking) experiences a dramatic brownout. This is not because he's a brute; it's just the wiring in his skull. Whether women experience a similar (*perhaps* less dramatic) brownout of brainpower after climaxing, the research I've seen doesn't say. But here's a more upbeat note: While the whole frontal cortex goes into la-la land, *one* area doesn't. This area, located in the right prefrontal cortex (tap your finger over your right eyebrow), goes *bonkers*. Yes, it's Orgasm Headquarters! It's as if all the other parts of the advanced brain sacrifice their power to create a momentary supernova explosion in Cum Towers.

Now here's a little kicker: This general area of the brain has also been found to get extremely excited while its owner is in the throes of artistic creation.

Art is like an orgasm without the moaning; an orgasm, like art without the easel. Lucky for you, you can enjoy both!

---

give him the
double oral door

18

When a woman is giving a man oral sex, most often she is the one in control. There's a reason for this: If the man is free to thrust into her mouth as he does into her vagina, and gets a little too excited, he could batter her tonsils. Yet, many men may find it very exciting to—once in a while—be the plunger rather than the plunged-down-upon.

Try this. She joins her hands together, with her thumbs crossed and her fingers intertwined, making him a little "vagina," which she moistens with her saliva. She holds her hands just in front of her mouth, and he goes through this first door into the second door of her mouth—over and over. She uses her hands to control him if he gets too rambunctious. If she's over him, she can also move her head up and down as required.

For an especially raunchy experience, she can lay back, her head on a couple of fluffy pillows while he straddles her and inserts his penis. She can tighten her hands to slow him down, if need be, while the pillows allow some strategic room for retreat.

roadblock remover #1
be more of a man without marlboros

19 Nearly everything in this book is positive—do this, try that. But sometimes the most truly positive—as in *effective*—step involves *not* doing something. Because no matter how much love you feel, no matter how enticing the lingerie, all may come to naught sexually because of certain roadblocks. There aren't many, but here's one.

Smoking. Okay, you already know it's bad for you, but the bad effect can hit a man's ability to have a firm erection before any other symptoms of circulatory damage show up. That's because the arteries that enter the penis are quite narrow, so any plaque and blockages can dramatically reduce blood flow.

If you have any doubts, consider this astonishing fact: At the Lahey Clinic for Sexual Function in Massachusetts, measurements were taken of the nighttime erections experienced by sleeping smokers who were impotent. These measurements are important, because if a man has nighttime erections, they signal that the problem is more or less fixable. When these men went without smoking for just one solitary day, the number of nighttime woodies went up by 40 percent!

doggy-style

20 One survey of thousands of men revealed that their number-one favorite position is doggy-style. For *them*, anyway. They seem to realize it isn't necessarily so great for their partners, because another survey found that forced to have sex in only one position from now until the end of time, twice as many would choose the woman-on-top than doggy-style.

With some new tricks, though, the doggy-style can be made more satisfying for the woman—and the man as well.

By the way, doggy-style is *not* anal sex; it's vaginal penetration from the rear instead of the front.

The classic approach is for the woman to support herself on her knees and hands as the man enters her. He is now in a position to either squeeze her butt or lean forward to fondle her breasts.

Two things about doggy-style, at this point. First, it allows for very deep penetration, which might feel good to the man, and possibly the woman, but his penis could end up banging against her cervix or bladder, which might not feel so good to her. Second, there tends to be little direct clitoral stimulation, so the man can reach around and provide some. If he doesn't, she can give him the idea by reaching down and doing it herself—if she can support herself with one hand.

Doggy-style *does* allow for intense stimulation of her G-spot, though, which can compensate for any shortcomings.

alcohol **as foreplay**

21

The publisher of a French magazine that reviews gourmet restaurants once said to me, "The reason the French like to drink wine is that we believe it facilitates social intercourse."

True enough. But wine facilitates *sexual* intercourse as well, doesn't it, André?

Which is strange when you think about it, because, as you probably know, alcohol is basically a depressant. Like other depressants, if taken in excessive amounts, it can make you unconscious, or worse. So why would wine facilitate *any* kind of intercourse?

Because, the first thing your merlot or Grey Goose depresses is the part of your brain that's packed with inhibitions. The inhibitions that depress any impulses you feel to forget about work, decorum, and caution, and just enjoy the hell out of yourself.

While alcohol, therefore, is a kind of biochemical foreplay, you have to be careful with it. Because after depressing your inhibitions, it could go to depressing other stuff. Like, oh, the penis, for instance. And, yes, the clitoris.

The average person's system can only detoxify about one drink per hour. If you drink faster than that, you begin to get bombed—bombed out of commission. And if you drink without eating anything, you get smashed all the faster, because food—especially protein and fats—slows down the absorption of alcohol. Cheese is a good slower-downer.

welcome to **my penis**

Most men will find any approach short of a finger-nail-snap a satisfactory how-do-you-do. There are some ways to be little more thoughtful, though. After the almost reflexive up-and-down hand slide, make this change: When the woman reaches the end of his stiffening stiffy, she turns her wrist over and descends thumb-down. Only the thumb shouldn't be pointing down; it'll jab him. Wrap the thumb around so it touches the forefinger. For some strange reason, having a woman do his penis this way feels especially good to a man. When she reaches the bottom, she changes hand position and comes up. From here on, it changes randomly—not knowing so simple a thing as which way her hand will be held next is exciting in itself.

When he is 99 percent hard, and not before then, she throws in some helmet straightening. That is, when her hand reaches the rim and head of his penis, she twists her hand as if she were trying to rotate it, while applying palm pressure to the very top. She makes a few circles, then descends again, and repeats in random patterns. For good luck, throw in a little flick of the tongue, aimed at the notch on the underside of his corona.

This is a reliable male warmer-upper, and can be intensified by other techniques, such as gentle scrotum pulling and twisting, or the hand action described under "Beyond Stroking—Way Beyond."

add a **sound track**

23

A great many men get off on hearing their partners make noises while they're making love. Probably because it makes them feel like they're pleasing you.

If issuing sighs, moans, and even screams is not your cup of tea, even when you're excited, take my advice—*try it anyway*. There's a reason that movies have sound tracks: It adds a whole other dimension to the story. Who knows, you may even get more excited yourself!

missionary position
upgrade #1

24

Put your hands under her hips, lifting them just slightly. Support your weight on your elbows. In this position you'll be a little higher, giving more stimulation to her clitoris. And your face will be closer to hers.

a man's intro to
buying her lingerie

25

Lingerie is a great traditional enhancement to your love life. It's sexy, but more: it's also romantic, looks great, feels great, and makes a fine gift on any occasion. If you are a man who feels intimidated by the thought of buying lingerie for your sweetheart, here's how to get your courage up.

The first thing you need to do is to find out her size, and if you want to surprise her, you can't ask. You'll have to sneak into her closet when she's not home, and check the size labels. Slight problem: These labels are likely to have numerical sizes (like 10) while most lingerie is sold in word sizes (medium). Here's your cheat sheet:

DRESS SIZE	LINGERIE SIZE
2–4	Extra Small
6–8	Small
10–12	Medium
14	Large
16–18	X-Large or 1X
20–22	2X
22–24	3X
24–26	4X

You are now ready to confidently enter a lingerie shop like Victoria's Secret and have a sales associate show you a bunch of options. You may find it more convenient to do your shopping on the Internet (and you'll find a wider range of sizes). Even if you do prefer a retail store, you may want to visit the Web first, so when the salesperson asks what you'd like to see, you won't have to answer, "Duhhhhh."

Three sites (among *many*) worth an introductory visit are *www.4everhers.com*, *www.hipsandcurves.com*, and *www.flirtylingerie.com*. Once you've learned the difference between a baby doll, a chemise, a teddy, and all the other styles, you're ready to poke around on any site or in any store.

A FEW TIPS: **When in doubt as to size, err on the large size. Check the return policy; panties, for instance, are usually not returnable. Always check for clearance sales; you can often buy perfectly fine lingerie for a fraction of what it would normally cost!**

Fantasy #1

"i will have you—now!"

26

Here we act out the very common fantasy of male dominance and female submission. And I mean *act*. There's a situation... a storyline... a *seamy* storyline. Pirate captures prim schoolteacher on her way to teach in the Caribbean. Bandito snares peasant girl bringing flowers to church. Hairy biker captures cyclist out for a training ride. The kind of story that they wouldn't show on HBO even at 2:00 A.M., because of the compulsion, which is forbidden after the first body parts are bared.

The man is going to rudely, lustfully, rip off her clothes. She struggles. But not all that much. Because her attacker, after all, is the guy she loves.

Not for everyone, perhaps, but the dominance-submission fantasy is extremely common, and giving yourself a chance to see what it feels like in the flesh, instead of just the mind, can be very, very hot.

erotic dishwashing

Many women, and I suppose some men, though I'm not one of them, don't feel comfortable about going upstairs for a roll in the hay while there are still unwashed pots, pans, dishes, and silverware—not to mention blenders, processors, shredders, and God knows what—strewn about the premises. The problem is that by the time all this stuff is gathered, washed, dried, stacked, and racked, the woman—who let's assume also cooked the meal—is too tired and mentally numbed for sex.

The solution, suggested to me by a woman friend, is so simple as to be shocking: Man does dishes; end of problem. When he does this, it's more than pitching in. It's a clear signal to his woman that he wants her body and soul and is willing to scrape off congealed cheese, wipe appliances that have 25 surfaces, and otherwise turn a mess into a home fit for great, carefree sex. With any luck, my friend explained, this chore could become a habit, which would only serve to increase the couple's intimacy and improve their love life. Or so she claims. She's probably right.

Now here's a tip for all you guys who decide to pitch in at clean-up time. Watch your wife carefully, and do the job exactly as she does—same soap, same kind of towel, same stacking technique, same putting-away spots for dry stuff. If you do it *one bit different* than she does, you will not lessen her discomfort about going upstairs, but increase it! I know whereof I speak.

> POSTSCRIPT: **Shortly after I wrote the above, an actual study came out from the University of California at Riverside, showing that women find men who do lots of chores around the house to be not only nice guys, but extremely sexually attractive!**

the incredible
22-step b.j.

28 The third-century Indian *Kama Sutra* (Book of Love) has a keen appreciation of teasing. The essence of the particular intimacy I will describe is, in fact, two-thirds teasing and just one-third pleasing—hence the high number of steps.

After each step, you see, the woman says something along the lines of "This is as far as I'm going tonight." The man then encourages, pleads, *begs* her to go on to the next step, which, in her good time, she does. The script, which I have adapted with a few modifications from the original ancient text (and you should feel free to change yourselves), goes like this:

The woman grasps the man with her hand, places his penis against her lips, and slowly takes the tip only into her mouth, with shallow in-and-out motions.

"That's all you get tonight."

"Oh, please, please!"

She nibbles—with her lips only—the sides of his head.

"I don't feel like doing any more than that."

"Please, sweetheart, please!"

She closes her lips tightly over the head of penis, and squeezes down.

"I think you're getting too excited."

"No, no! It's wonderful!"

She takes his penis a little deeper into her mouth, again gives the head a squeezing kiss, then spits it out, saying:

"That's enough for one night."

"Please, more, *more*!"

She takes his penis in her hand, turns her wrist so her thumb is pointing down (but wrapped around to touch her forefinger) and slides her grip down slowly, with very firm pressure. Then she reverses hand position and comes up, just barely touching him. Repeat half a dozen times or more, as desired.

"Haven't you had enough yet?"

"No, I want more! Please, give it to me! Let me feel your mouth again!"

She licks his entire penis with the tip of her tongue, then once again takes his head into her mouth for intimate licks.

"I'm getting tired. I'm going to stop."

"You can't stop! I'll die!"

She once again takes his penis into her mouth, applying pressure with her lips. When it is halfway in, she sucks on it hard, as if sucking the sweet juice from an orange or mango. Then she releases it and holds it so the tip skims over her lips.

"You've had all you're going to get. You don't want to come on my face, do you?"

"Yes! I mean, *no!* You can't stop now! Take me, *take all of me!*"

With her man nearly mad with desire, she swallows his penis as deeply as she can, using her lips to tighten her grip, and her tongue to rub against the underside. He moans. She moans. He comes, and she allows his semen to splash on her lips, chin, or cheeks. Finally, she rubs his penis head gently along her lips, and takes a lick or two.

why a divorce
is good for you

"You can never be happily married until you get a divorce from yourself."—Jerry McCant

The same goes for a happy sexual relationship. While it's important to seek your own satisfaction, the truth is that if you regard everything that goes on between you only in terms of your own pleasure, you ain't gonna get that much pleasure over the long haul.

In a good relationship, partners make choices together about what they're going to do or not do. They not only accommodate their partners, but go out of their way to please and delight the other. You may still have the Me Generation thing going on in your head, but if you let it take charge in bed, your sex life will be only a fraction of what it would be in the Us Generation.

sex toys 101

30

It's easy to imagine that most people who use sex toys (like vibrators) are sexually frustrated, turning to technology for want of an eager lover. That idea is totally false, however. Surveys show that people who use sex toys have sex (with members of the opposite gender) more often than those who wouldn't know sex toys from Legos.

Another misconception is that sex toys, even when used with a lover, somehow replace or disenfranchise your partner. In truth, the use of various sex toys can be a very mutual, intimate practice. It says, "I trust you to do something that many other people regard as weird." Further, it permits the partners to learn a lot more about how they can please and satisfy each other, by seeing how they react to various sensations in different places.

You might also have the notion that sex toys are cheaply made pieces of crap, because no one is going to try to return a vibrator. I sort of suspected that myself. But I soon discovered that nearly all the sex toys I purchased online were, in fact, of very high, even outstanding quality. Prices tend to be lower than what you'd expect, too. And the goods arrive at your home in tasteful, we-can-keep-a-secret packaging.

There's another thing I really like about sex toys. When you first open the package and look at them, they often make you chuckle. Laugh at loud. Or gasp. Why? Because many are fiendishly clever, and some simply shockingly large. Opening your sex toys with your partner creates an atmosphere of "This is a hoot! Wait'll I use this on you!" That lightens things up a lot, if they need lightening, and creates the proper feeling of experimentation and mutual adventure.

Just one more thing: Sex toys can be used as pure enhancements to sex, providing sensations you couldn't experience otherwise (unless, for instance, a man has AA batteries in his scrotum), but also as aids, providing for things such as spot-on clitoral stimulation, that can make strong orgasm a near certainty as opposed to "maybe this time."

Please keep this in mind as you read further on, and we describe various toys. At least *trying* a few can be both insanely pleasurable and an honest-to-goodness mind-opening experience at the same time.

---

a bedroom
boner

31

Some women delight in creating a Victorian boudoir. Mauve and pink flowered prints on the bedspread and draperies; piles of tufted pillows with ruffles and bows; velvet upholstery; lace doilies on the dressers and tables; silk flowers; candles...maybe even a four-poster bed. Such a look stirs her romantic juices: She puts one bare foot on the parquet floor and she's ready for love.

But some men instantly imagine they have been led into a showroom at Ovarian Reflections. Consciously or unconsciously, they feel like they don't belong there, and so does their dingdorum.

Now, many guys will not find such a boudoir off-putting. They may even find it a definite turn-on to be entering a woman's private lair. Not sure how your man feels? Ask him if he thinks it's too feminine; if he would enjoy a different sort of hormone vibe in the bedroom décor.

He *would?* Now what? We're not saying that you should take the framed needlepoint off the wall and replace it with a moose head. But do *something.* A full-length mirror is a pretty style-neutral fixture that many men will find enjoyably provocative. Nineteenth-century prints featuring manly dogs like setters or Newfoundlands, rugged landscapes, game birds, or sleek sailboats cutting through white-caps are all good choices. Bullfighter posters, however, are pretty much out of the question style-wise.

There's another option: Go all the way with the Victoriana theme. Specifically, wear black, lacy, provocative lingerie, the kind that goes with your *décor d'amore*, as you enter the bedroom. Undress slowly.

ebruary

the joy
of the g-spot

1 The G-Spot is named for Dr. Ernst Grafenberg, who described and popularized it years ago, though non-European authorities already knew as much centuries before he got around to it. In any case, the G-Spot is usually described as a dime-size area located a few inches into the vagina on the front, or outer, wall. Actually, it isn't in the vagina per se, but just outside it, though, especially when aroused, it can be felt as a rough spot by an exploring finger. And, when aroused, it "inflates" both in value and size from a dime to a quarter.

Not every woman will find her G-spot to be a tremendous turn-on when rubbed against, but many will. Teaching your lover to find it isn't difficult. Barbara Keesling, Ph.D., suggests that he holds his hand palm up and inserts his index finger straight into her vagina. When it's all the way in, he curls back his finger as if motioning "Come 'ere!" His fingertip will then be pointing at her pubic mound. He then slowly moves his finger around, and with any luck, she'll become excited, which he may note by sensing the spot becoming swollen and even pulsing.

The best intercourse position for stimulating the G-spot is any variation of doggy-style. Whatever position the man is in, he can usually apply more pressure to it by simply pointing his penis toward the woman's navel.

believe it or not #1
the pussy snorkel

2 When seriously and deeply into giving his woman oral sex, a man sometimes has trouble breathing. That's especially true if the woman has her legs wrapped around his head...even more so if the act is taking place underwater.

Enter the Pussy Snorkel. This device has short little tubes that fit into a man's nose, connected to hoses that fit behind his head. Aside from allowing him to breathe more easily, the snorkel also does away with any problems in the vaginal odor department. There's a bonus here for the recipient: A small clitoral stimulator on the other side of the breathing apparatus!

FOR MORE INFORMATION: **www.lingerietoys.inadult.com.**

fantasy #2
super bowl sex

3 SUPER BOWL SUNDAY

If you want him to peel his eyes off the TV screen and check your field position, one surefire way is to get yourself a saucy cheerleader's outfit. The best we've seen, by far, is the Dallas Cheerleader's costume, with a stylish, low-cut blue top; tight, skimpy blue-and-white shorts with a gold tassel; and of course, pom-poms. Besides doing your cheerleader routine, you should also try some player actions: illegal backfield motion, for instance, or even intentional grounding. By halftime, you may be forced to put up a goal line stand.

FOR MORE INFORMATION: **www.threewisheslingerie.com.**

her turn **to churn**

4 You may remember the "churning" technique described last month, wherein the man inserts the head of his penis, holds the shaft, and moves it round and round. Here's the female version of the same idea.

She sits on him, face-to-face, takes in his already-ready penis, closes her legs firmly around him, and then moves her hips in a circular motion as if churning butter.

---

r-e-s-p-e-c-t!

5 Aretha Franklin's hit record isn't just a classic erotic love song; it's also terrific advice. Therapist John Gottman, Ph.D., and colleagues conducted an intensive study of relationship intricacies among couples and concluded that "Respect is one of the greatest aphrodisiacs."

This seems to be a novel concept. *Respect* as a turn-on? When we show respect in church, say, by not chatting, yawning, or furtively using our cell phones, I doubt that Father McManus or anyone else is aroused. At least, I hope not. The funny—or sad—thing is, we often fail to show respect for the person that means the most to us. Not listening when they talk, always doubting their judgment, underrating their intelligence, ignoring their friends or family, and not making them feel appreciated are common ways we fail to deliver what Aretha demands. Even if we sincerely love them, failing to show that love when they walk in the door after a day at work, for instance, is disrespectful.

Now turn all these failings into positives, and you not only improve your relationship but also, as the good doctor suggests, your sex life.

---

the exterior
french kiss

Lou Paget, esteemed author of *The Big O*, suggests that you can add an erotic touch to kissing by taking hold of your lover's lower lip (with your lips, or gently with your teeth) and then using the tip of your tongue to titillate him just under his outer lip. Theoretically, this tiny spot is very sensitive. Make sure he's shaved closely beforehand! Licking the inside of your lover's *upper* lip is another nice variation.

mutual **bondage**

7

This is not about your investments; it's about a whole dimension of sexual fun and excitement that you may not yet have explored.

I call it mutual bondage instead of bondage or restraint or sexual power play (all terms used by different folks) to emphasize that this is a mutual act that both partners agree to and enjoy. And, of course, it does involve some degree of bondage or restraint, though always on the safe and nonharmful side. What's more, it must also be accompanied by mutual respect, mutual care, and clear communication.

You might wonder, what, exactly, mutual bondage has to do with "normal" sex? You'd be surprised!

First, a poll of readers of *Glamour* magazine revealed that some 29 percent of respondents said their number-one favorite sex fantasy was *not* having sex wearing a $12,000 gown, *not* having sex while dancing with a prince in his castle, and *not* with Russell Crowe in his dressing room during a break in the filming of *Pride and Prejudice: The Honeymoon*. No, it was having sex while being restrained.

Second, another survey concluded that half of all men fantasize about being the "dominator" during sex. The same percentage of women fantasize about being dominated, the survey found.

Third, approximately 70 percent of both women and men fantasize while having sex. While the core of the drama unfolding in the men's minds is "conquest," the theme of women's fantasies revolves around "active surrender", according to Helen Fisher, Ph.D., in her book *Why We Love*.

These are not rape fantasies, Dr. Fisher declares. In "active surrender," the woman feels that there is some degree of compulsion, but she also finds it extremely exciting and pleasurable. Likewise, a man who wants to use some means of compulsion, be it physical or psychological, imagines that the woman is actually more than willing, even if she won't openly admit it, to find enjoyment in his arms.

The research I've seen doesn't say much about the number of *men* who enjoy the experience of being sexually dominated. My guess is that many do. Likewise, I believe many women get a big kick out of being the dominator. Switching roles is, as I see it, a big and exciting part of mutual bondage.

Mutual bondage, keep in mind, is play-acting. It's not about venting your feelings of anger or jealousy or anything like that. If you are, in fact, angry with your lover, that is not the time for mutual bondage.

Most important of all: When two people agree to be restrained, bound, teased, tickled, or "ordered" to give or receive certain sex acts, it requires a very high degree of trust. That in itself can be deeply arousing and can raise your level of intimacy to a higher—albeit different—level. Keep that in mind as you read later about various ways of enjoying mutual bondage.

watching the world's
sexiest movies

8

Not sex movies—we'll talk about them later—but suggestive, erotic, or downright steamy movies. Nearly everyone enjoys them, and they certainly can put you in the mood, if not the nude. Here is a sampling of what people tell me they think are the best:

Better Than Chocolate, 9½ Weeks, Dangerous Liaisons, Body Heat, The Postman Always Rings Twice, The Pillow Book, Last Tango in Paris, Tie Me Up, Tie Me Down, Henry and Jane, Baby Doll, Holy Smoke, and *Wild Things.* Try these or have fun finding the ones that work for you and your partner.

---

sweeten your sex life
with chocolate

9

Magazines and books are forever stating that chocolate is a "love food" because it contains a chemical called PEA (phenylethylamine) that stimulates an area of the brain associated with feelings of love. This is an enchanting notion, especially around Valentine's Day. It's also almost certainly false.

Chocolate doesn't actually contain that much PEA to begin with. Second, when some researchers gorged on chocolate for days and then measured PEA levels in their urine, they found no change at all. It appears as though any PEA we eat is blast-metabolized by the body into other stuff, and doesn't add to the complement of PEA our bodies produce. While eating anything sweet and fatty will cause the brain's pleasure centers to begin twinkling a bit brighter, it seems that chocolate has no more "love potion" power than, say, salami (which also contains PEA.)

Okay, so chocolate is not the prince's kiss on the sleeping maiden of love. But, ... it could well be the French kiss on the sleeping maiden of sex.

Recent research in universities and medical centers has shown that chocolate—not cheap milk chocolate, but really dark chocolate—has a dramatic beneficial effect on the flow of blood through arteries. Poor blood flow—remember that the penile arteries are very narrow—is the chief cause of potency problems in men, and is now believed to be a major problem for many not-so-young-anymore women.

One study at the University of California at San Francisco showed that eating a 1.5-ounce bar of Dove Dark chocolate (known to be rich in the beneficial compounds called flavanols) brought about a surge of available nitric oxide, the "muscle" compound needed for artery dilation. And yes, the arteries did dilate more—about 10 percent more.

More recently, researchers at the Athens Medical School in

Greece used larger chocolate bars—3.5-ounce extra dark bars—then ran ultrascans on the people who ate them. They found better blood flow for the next 3 hours and better functioning of the arterial endothelial cells that prevent plaque buildup and fight high blood pressure. One of the Greek cardiologists in the study says the compounds in the chocolate also increased levels of our old friend nitric oxide.

More recent research shows that dark chocolate tends to raise "good" HDL cholesterol. Chocolate has also been shown to reduce blood platelet aggregation, the same benefit conferred by low-dose aspirin.

With all this, it's not so surprising that a long-term study of Harvard grads found that confessed chocoholics were outliving those who never touched the stuff.

Most of the chocolate we see on the shelves of food markets and snack bars is not the kind used in these experiments. At present, the Mars candy people, who make Dove Dark products, pretty much have a lock on the best stuff. And they probably deserve it, because they've been doing R&D in the field for 15 years. Seems that the flavanol levels in chocolate are affected by all sorts of things, from the region where the cocoa beans are grown, to how the beans are fermented, roasted, shipped, and so on. Mars uses a "Cocoapro" logo on products that meet their standards for high levels of flavanols.

By the way, even really expensive, really dark chocolate candies can be not very good; the creamy butters and sugar they're filled with don't have enough of the "right stuff."

If eating 1 to 3 ounces of chocolate on a regular basis seems likely to frighten your bathroom scale, you're right. The chocolate bars consumed in the classic tests had some 200 calories each. Besides their Dark Chocolate Singles bars, Dove also has Dark Chocolate Promises, which have just 42 calories each, but you'd have to eat five to get into the serious health-boosting range. That might not be difficult to achieve. But remember, since gaining weight might well cancel the health effect, you must reduce the calories in the rest of your diet by the same amount of calories contained in the chocolate. Many people will find that eliminating other sweets, cookies, and chips is enough to do the trick.

If your store doesn't carry Dove products, a good alternative, especially for baking, is the semi-sweet baking bars made by Ghirardelli.

---

the better sex
chocolate walnut brownie

10

The latest news on the chocolate front comes from Italy, where researchers have discovered that *women who eat chocolate on a regular basis have more sex drive—and sexual satisfaction—than women who don't.* I think that fact deserves italics, don't you?

Now, you might imagine that chocolate-lovers are simply more pleasure-oriented, and so would be more likely to find enjoyment in sex, but in light of all the other research showing that chocolate physically improves circulation, I think there's at least some cause-and-effect going on here. Enough, at least, for a better-sex chocolate recipe, complete with walnuts, which, as we noted before, are also rich in compounds that boost sex drive and performance.

The following recipe was the winner in a taste test we held; it's adapted from Sharon Moore's fine little book, *Brownies.*

CHOCOLATE WALNUT BROWNIES

5 ounces unsweetened chocolate
½ cup unsalted butter
4 large eggs
2 cups sugar

1 teaspoon vanilla extract
1 cup all-purpose flour
¼ teaspoon salt
1 cup chopped walnuts

Preheat oven to 350F. Lightly grease an 8" square baking pan and set aside.

Melt the chocolate and butter in a double boiler, or in a heavy-bottomed pan, over low heat.

In a large mixing bowl, beat the eggs well. Beat in the sugar and vanilla. Blend in the melted chocolate mixture, then fold in flour, salt, and walnuts.

Pour into the pan and spread evenly, then bake for about 25 minutes. Let cool, then cut into squares—or use a cookie cutter to cut into hearts!

makeup **sex**

11

I'd bet every long-time couple knows at least one secret they don't teach in sex-ed: Sex that follows "making up" after a fight is often incredible. I'd also bet that some couples *purposely* get into spats (consciously or not) to spice up their sex lives.

Getting into a fight causes testosterone to spike in both people, and testosterone is a sex-drive potion for both men and women, points out Helen Fisher, Ph.D. When you have sex just after the fight is over, but your testosterone doesn't yet realize it, you are body surfing in a big wave of warm hormones.

This is not to suggest fighting as foreplay. But if you do squabble, the important thing is to make up before you go to sleep, or else the deal is off.

enhancing your **pubic décor**

12

According to research reported in the red-blooded magazine *Men's Health*, guys have some decided opinions about pubic hair—at least when it's on a woman.

First off, 40 percent of men would actually prefer if their partners shaved off all their hair. I'm not sure why this is, though my research department suggests it could be because many women of the night and porn stars shave themselves, and some guys find this a naughty turn-on. If you disdain any and all trimming, and just let your bush grow where and how it pleases, be aware that only one man in 20 approves of such.

Most surprising is that 27 percent of guys told the pollsters that they'd like to see their woman's pubic hair "sculpted like a topiary." A topiary, just in case you don't now, is a sizeable shrubbery that has been carved and trimmed to take on an unnatural shape, like a cone or an egg—or sometimes, even an animal: a bunny for instance.

Should this idea appeal to you—and I just *know* it does—you might consider a heart shape, higher in the center than the edges for that sculpted look. Or a butterfly, perhaps. One of my female advisors suggested a penis-shaped topiary, with the ridge of the head higher than the rest. Use your imagination, but under no circumstance create a sculpture that resembles a beaver.

Bikini trimmers, made for shaving pubic hair, are available at such sites as *www.boots.com* and *www.remingtonproducts.com*.

for valentine's day
burn a hunk o' love

13

For lovers, Valentine's Day is kind of like Easter, Yom Kippur, and Thanksgiving rolled into one. And, holy cow, it's tomorrow, so hopefully, you're reading this ahead of time!

If you already know what you'll buy (or make) your love, congratulations! If not, here's a suggestion that may intrigue you. Burn her or him a CD of special love songs, the songs that touch your heart and perhaps have a special meaning to you as a couple. After you "burn" your collection (if you don't know how, check your software manual) you can slip a photo of the two of you into the cover, and a list of songs on the back cover of the case.

For what it's worth, here are a few of the songs I included in my Valentine's album: *In the Midnight Hour* by Wilson Pickett, *Warm and Tender Love* by Percy Sledge, *In My Life* by the Beatles, *Hunk o' Burnin' Love* by The King, and *Kokomo* by the Beach Boys.

Sappy, huh? What are *your* favorites?

be "the apprentice"
for valentine's day

14 VALENTINE'S DAY

Offering to be your lover's slave for a day is a good idea, but this is better. An "apprentice," as you know if you've watched the TV show, doesn't just do what she or he is ordered to do, but uses creativity, imagination, and every personal resource to make the greatest positive impression.

So on Valentine's Day (and perhaps her birthday), tell her in advance—so she has time to dream up her wish list—that you will do anything and everything she wants you to. From making breakfast, doing chores, repairs, shopping trips, cooking and serving dinner, having a conversation on any desired subject, and of course, romantic and sexual wishes, your goal is to make her feel like the Queen of the Nile.

Throw in as many extra touches as you can. If she wants a foot rub, first wash her feet in warm, soapy, scented water. Put rose petals in her path. Write a love note and slip it under her dinner plate. Buy her a present, like sultry lingerie. Prepare for a night of romantic love, with aromatic candles, a massage, and the all the trimmings for a long, beautiful night of passion

With any luck, she'll say to you, just before she nods off: "You're *hired*."

mount your
racehorse

15

From a fragment of an ancient Greek book on sex that has survived the ages, scholars know that folks like Mr. and Mrs. Aristotle were fond of a position called *keles*—which translates as "racehorse." They also have discovered through their scholarly efforts that it involved the woman being on top, facing his head, in the same position she'd be in if she were riding the man as if he were a spirited steed.

This position is best done when the man is erect and ready to accept the weight of his rider. Her knees will probably be along his sides, though she could try straightening them as well. From her bareback saddle, she can rise up and down, or lean backwards, imagining, if she wishes, that her horse is in a kind of slow-motion gallop.

If the woman is really into equestrianism, she can whip her steed with a length of silken cord, urging him to do her bidding. You might even want to give him a name, like Man o' War or Sea Biscuit.

red river, **blue sky**

16

Some women feel uneasy about having sex during their periods. Some men do, too. But once you get past worrying about stains on sheets and thighs, you may be surprised at the possible bonus waiting. At least one sex therapist says that the dramatic hormone shifts that accompany menstruation can cause many women to want more, not less, sex at this time.

---

shock sex #1
say the forbidden word

17

Most often we think of putting someone in the mood for sex as involving candlelight dinners or languorous massage. But there is another way—the exact opposite. An approach so unexpected, so brazen, that it hits the other person like an electric charge.

Here is one that certainly worked on me: As I sat there immersed in piles of work, ignoring my partner, she sat down across the table from me and said these unforgettable words: *"How'd you like to go upstairs for a little c...sucking?"* It was the greatest, most exciting idea I'd ever heard, especially coming from the mouth of a woman who seldom uses any naughty language. Funny how a four-letter word can have more erotic appeal than a four-poster bed—to men anyway!

Next time your man is ignoring you, and you're in the mood, try Shock Sex #1 and see how it works. By the way, if any readers find this technique too tawdry for their taste, they are advised not to read the Shock Sex tips that come later, 'cause some are worse.

---

pronouns and **sex**

18 When you are saying something *positive* to your lover, always start with "you." "You're so beautiful." "You're so hot." "You're so hard."

When saying something of a *corrective* nature to your lover, always begin with "I." "I like it when you do that faster" (instead of "You're going too slow"). "I'm getting sore there" (instead of "You're hurting me"). "I'm getting soft" (instead of "You're not *doing* anything!").

please,
take my hand

19 That's the refrain in one of the 3,000 old R&B songs that are canoeing around in my brain. It's also the refrain of many sex therapists, though, because "hand-in-hand" is perhaps the most basic—but often forgotten—learning techniques in the school for better sex.

Whichever partner is the least hesitant holds out a hand and invites the other to place his or hers over theirs. She (I'm assuming the woman goes first) then slowly and deliberately places her hand on those parts of her body that appreciate manual attention. And not just the *where*, but the *how*, too. There will probably be an instinct to begin with those areas that she likes touched first, and gradually move on to the more intense pleasure venues. As his hand rides over hers, he feels all the pressure changes, rhythms, directions, twists and turns, and little tricks that she appreciates.

Then he puts his hand *under* hers and goes back to point A. He tries his best to mimic what she showed him, as she patiently tutors him with her top-riding hand. She may also give him little gold stars with appropriate soft moaning sounds.

The beloved Charlie Brown, as he lay in bed, once asked, "Where have I gone wrong?"

A voice answered him, saying "This is going to take more than one night."

And yes, this is going to take more than one night, too. Be patient. Be rewarding. It's worth the effort, believe me. And what the hay—it's fun!

Now it's his turn to let her hand ride on his. Yes, I know what you're thinking: He doesn't have to bother. He can just *point*.

Well, that's not true. There are more things a man wants to feel than a hand clasped around his Titan rocket. He may, for instance, like little circles made around his nipples. A finger drawn slowly and teasingly down his abdomen. On his penis, different strokes that his partner might never have imagined he likes. Little finger moves, squeezes. His testicles played with or gently pulled. Rolling over on his side, he might also want to show her what he'd like done on his butt. Love and learn.

the sex power food
for the older man

20

As recently as 10 years ago, nutritionists rarely recommended blueberries, favoring the likes of strawberries, oranges, and melons as sources of vitamins. Now that we know that vitamins are only part of the health promoters in foods, blueberries have suddenly come into their own. Speaking of coming...

"Blueberries are one of the best foods for older men with erectile problems," states Mary Ellen Camire, Ph.D., a professor of food science. The reason is that the little blue boys are loaded with natural compounds that relax blood vessels and improve circulation.

I usually put my blueberries on top of cereal. Lately, I've been eating a high-fiber cereal, which has tons of fiber but only about a gram of taste, so the blueberries make it infinitely more edible.

You can also eat a bowl of blueberries mixed with blackberries, strawberries, or other fruit as a great snack. If (again, like me) you use low-fat milk, add that to the fruit bowl. You can make it especially inviting by mixing one-third fat-free half-and-half in with your milk.

---

sex with a
sore back

21

Muscle spasms are not a good lead-in to love spasms, so if the man has a sore back, try this doctor-recommended approach.

She lies on her stomach, on a low bed (or low piece of furniture). Her legs are on the floor, her butt at the edge of the bed. The man enters her, leans forward cautiously, and places his elbows by her sides, to take pressure off his back. As he somewhat gingerly moves back and forth, he makes most of the motion with his legs, instead of dirty-dancing pelvic thrusts.

Find my honey, honey

22

Put dabs of honey on the parts of your body you want your lover to lick and suck. Don't tell him or her where they are. Hide at least one little dab someplace like in your ear or in between your toes.

roadblock remover #2
turn fat into love muscle

23 Chubby Hubby is more than a Ben & Jerry's flavor. It's a major cause of sexual difficulties, even impotence. (While overweight may not affect women with the same dramatic problems, it often causes psychological problems, like simple embarrassment, that diminish the enjoyment of sex.) One factor is that overweight tends to interfere with healthy blood flow.

But here's something few people realize: Fat men have an insidious tendency to turn testosterone into estrogen—to become hormonally feminized, in other words. Obviously, this can't do him (or her) any good. What does do good is losing the weight. Tests show that nearly all men who lose a significant amount of weight feel more sexual desire, and about one-third actually enjoy better sexual function. Of course, they don't measure *that* at the famous Weight Watchers weigh-ins, but, hey, maybe they *should!*

the world's most
pleasing vibrator

24

Often labeled the Wascally Rabbit, this vibrator is, at least as I write this, the number-one selling penislike vibrator in the known universe. There are several good reasons for its popularity.

Its exterior—all 7-plus inches of it—is formed from soft "jelly" plastic, which gives a softer, gentler feel than hard plastic. That's good, because this baby is pretty big, with a head nearly 5 inches in circumference. The rabbit part juts out from the base, angled in such a way as to provide direct stimulation to the clitoris. The rabbit, including both its ears, vibrates either with the shaft or alone, under separate controls. Yes! In the middle of the shaft is a ball of visible beads that rock and roll along with the vibes. And if that's not enough, the tip of the vibrator actually *rotates in circles!*

The unit that controls speed is attached by a coiled white cord, and can be operated by either partner.

This sex toy, or one like it, was featured in a very funny episode of *Sex and the City*; that may be one reason it's so popular. Our own research found it well-deserving of its success: In a word, it's *fantastic*.

> NOTE: **We bought ours at www.shop.sextoys.sex-superstore.com, but they're widely available.**

yet another reason
to snack on walnuts

25 We mentioned before that L-arginine, an amino acid, is the only food substance known to increase a woman's sex drive, and that walnuts are one of the best sources. Proving that there *is* a Cosmic Plan, after all, it turns out that walnuts can also do great things for a man's sex life.

Spanish medical researchers recently gave two groups of men similar heart-healthy diets that varied in only one factor. One group was given 8 to 13 walnuts a day (about 2 ounces). After just 1 month, the walnut-eaters had 20 percent less gunk in their arteries, and an incredible 64 percent stronger artery-pumping action. That could easily translate into much greater potency for a middle-aged man and better sex for women, too.

Why are walnuts so healthy? Two reasons.

One, the L-arginine—the component that makes a woman sexier—also acts as a raw material from which the body produces nitric oxide, an important vasodilator, or artery-opener.

Two, walnuts are the only nut (and one of the few nonfish foods of any kind) that contain good amounts of omega-3 fatty acids, which improve the functioning of people's nerves in such a way that makes them less hostile and mistrustful.

Walnuts: No boudoir should be without them!

smooth **moves**

26

Even if you've never used a lubricant before, it's a good idea to try one. Things go better, and often feel better, too. With sex toys, they're almost always needed, and with anal sex, always. Water-based lubes are recommended because they don't react with condoms or sex toys, don't cause problems in the vagina, and supposedly don't stain the sheets (try some on an old tee shirt to see if it does or doesn't). There are special, thicker lubes formulated specifically for anal sex.

Astroglide and Slippery Stuff are both poplar and often recommended. Sex therapist Lou Paget has her own favorites: Sensua, Sex Grease, Very Private Intimate Moisturizer, Liquid Silk, and Midnight Fire (which becomes warm on the skin).

Fire and ice **part 1**

27

Men, this is the only practical use you will ever make of your lady's tea cozy, I guarantee you. Brew up some tea in the cozy—which is designed, of course, to keep it good and hot for a long time—and put it on a tray.

Next to it place one empty glass (for the tea) and another glass filled with three-quarters ice and one-quarter water. Carry said tray to the bedroom. No, you are not going to drink tea in bed; not exactly, anyway.

When the moment comes that you are about to pleasure her with your tongue, take a sip of tea. Be careful not to burn yourself; that would ruin everything. Then, immediately apply your hot tongue to her clitoris. When the heat dissipates, as it soon will, take a sip of ice water. Go back to work. Tea, her, ice water, her; tea, her, ice water, her.

This drives most women wild, though some could be freaked out. If the latter proves to be the case, just drink the damn tea.

---

the reverse
racehorse

28

In the "racehorse" position, the woman is sitting upright, astride the man. Here, she is facing his feet, rather than his face. As she moves about in the saddle, up and down and forward and back, her G-spot should get more stimulation. The "reverse racehorse" might also be a good idea for women who would rather not be looking their steed in the eye.

march

more testosterone
by the spoonful

1 Besides sticking to your ribs (but not your waist!) and having all the other healthful qualities it's known for, oatmeal has a peculiar quality that Quaker Oats has not yet gotten around to brandishing on their boxes.

It's great for sex!

Seems that oats contain a substance that doesn't exactly produce testosterone, but rather frees up what you already have, and sends it sailing on its merry way throughout your body. Since testosterone is vital for the generation of sexual desire and performance in both men *and* women, and millions are now known to be short of this hormone, oatmeal deserves our hearty thanks.

To make oatmeal a bit more sensuous in the eating, try adding some fat free half-and-half to your milk.

> **BONUS:** Oatmeal also helps reduce cholesterol, and the lower your cholesterol, the less likely you are to have sexual dysfunction.

no-brainer #1
make bedtime co-ed

2 Sex therapists say that more couples are having dramatically less sex than they used to, and not because they have some sort of sexual dysfunction. It's more like a *mal* function—they simply aren't getting together, often because of mutually long, tough schedules.

One way this malfunction is exacerbated is the habit of not going to bed at the same time. When one trots off to the bedroom, the partner is still reading, watching TV, even working. While I suspect this is sometimes done as a sly means of avoiding sex, in many cases, it's just a really bad habit couples fall into. If so, *stop it!* Yes, it's a no-brainer, but the solutions to many problems are pretty obvious, don't you think?

missionary position
upgrade #2

3 This begins with the missionary position (funny how missionaries are better remembered today for their sexual proclivities than for their conversions!) but slips and slides into something different.

The man, astride his lady (this is the missionary position, remember), helps her raise one leg. Together, they both slowly roll until they are face-to-face on their sides, and they make love. There are several advantages to this orientation, according to Whit Barry, in his book *Making Love: A Man's Guide*. One is that the man isn't crushing the breath out of his woman. Nor is he getting tired supporting himself on his knees and elbows (good news for overweight or arthritic "missionaries"). Plus, he says, you will find this position engenders a kind of "cozy intimacy."

post-orgasmic
sex

4 Most, if not all of us, think of sex as ending with climax. If there's anything after that, it's classified as "afterglow." But perhaps this is more cultural than factual. Here is an excerpt from the ancient Indian love classic, *Kama Sutra* (The Book of Love), that puts a different glow on afterglow:

"Sometimes they [the lovers, following intercourse] sit on the rooftop porch to enjoy the moonlight, and tell stories that suit their mood. As she lies in his lap, looking at the moon, he points out the rows of constellations to her; they look at the Pleiades, the Pole Star, and the garland of Seven Sages that form the Great Bear. That is the end of sex."

Notice the author doesn't say "the end of afterglow" or "the end of romance," but "the end of *sex*." Clearly he has a more holistic view of what sex is all about than most of us!

So, perhaps we should pay more attention to the post-orgasmic part of sex. If you aren't good at pointing out constellations (I don't think I could locate the "Seven Sages" even if the Eighth Sage were sitting on my lap!), you could "tell stories that suit your mood." And, perhaps by the time this book is published, there will be an Astronomy Channel you can watch in bed!

john henry **sex**

5 John Henry was the famous steel-drivin' man who died with his hammer in his hand while pounding railroad spikes into the ground. John Henry is also what I call the sexual technique of hammering the penis straight down into the vagina (though I haven't written a folk song about this yet).

Though there are many other techniques, there's nothing wrong with being a John Henry. Often, in fact, it gets the job done like nothing else. But here's one tip for all you steel-drivin' men. Instead of whoppin' your hammer down like John Henry does in the song, and bringing it slowly back up, do the exact opposite. Go in slowly—take about 5 seconds—and withdraw it quickly. This will probably be a novel sensation for both, and it should give her clitoris a special charge.

Try it and see how it feels. At least, I doubt that you'll die with your hammer in your hand, like John Henry.

they don't sell
this ring
at tiffany's

6 It's called a cock ring, and there is no other name for it, unless you want to call it a penile constriction band, which sounds like a torture device instead of a sex aid. A man who wants firmer erections slips the ring on near the base of his penis, and as his penis expands, the ring cuts down on the amount of blood flowing back into the nonpenis part of his body. It works because the arteries carrying blood into the penis are in the central portion, and unaffected by the ring, while one of the veins carrying the blood out of the penis is close enough to the skin to be constricted by the "C"-word ring. Some rings are adjustable, which is obviously helpful. Some even *vibrate*, which may be good for both partners.

Of course, you can't keep these things on forever; you may not get gangrene, but you could get black and blue.

make candlelight
even better

7

Everyone knows that candlelight is somehow romantic. One author says it makes human skin look "more fluid and smooth." I tested this by looking at skin under both candlelight and lamplight and found it to be absolutely true.

I further discovered that taking off my reading glasses has pretty much the same effect. Both together—candles and no glasses—is nearly miraculous. Every little blemish, wrinkle, pore, and freckle is gone, replaced with a kind of liquid glow. It's like a fabulous makeup and lighting job you pull off in seconds.

---

james bond **sex**

8

This is an interesting and rather unusual technique that, for some quirky reason, I imagine James Bond often employed with his countless lovers, many of whom were spies and double agents. That may say more about me than Bond, but remember, fantasy is important!

Bond is sitting astride his woman, her legs atop his. With his manly assistance, she crosses over one of her legs so that the back of her thigh is against his chest. Turning a bit toward the side her lifted leg is coming from, he enters her. It's sort of a halfway house between front and rear entry...just the sort of thing that would appeal to an international spy! And Bond, no doubt, would make good use of his hands, as in massaging her secret pleasure button. Try this and see if you think 007 was into something good.

spike your love
with stiletto heels

Everyone knows that men find high spike heels very provocative. Whether that's because it's a cultural thing or because wearing high heels changes the shape of a woman's calves into a curve that's more flattering, is hard to say. But if casual, practical, comfortable shoes are all you ever wear, you're missing out on a chance to give him (and yes, maybe you, too) a special "wow" response when he checks you out.

Classic pumps, the kind you could wear to any party, are just the beginning. There's the popular platform look, complete with super-high heels to match. Shoes that show your whole foot, others with lots of leather or vinyl—even marabou. Sexy, long leg wraps that go to your calves. If you're into the dominatrix thing, there are long black shoes that go up well over the knee, with long sexy openings on the side. That particular number is called, simply, "Ferocious." Not made by Rockport. Collections of erotic footwear can be seen at *www.lingeriesite.com* and *www.trashy.com*.

Fire and ice
part two

10 The same hot tea/ice water protocol we described for exciting her clitoris can also be tried on her nipples. Here is a much simpler way of achieving a similar effect. Wet the tips of your fingers in your mouth and touch her nipples. Then blow on them.

hard as a **rock**

11 That's because it *is* a rock. A rock dildo, to be precise. And not just any rock, either, but handcrafted granite. The Twist Stone Dildo has a rounded head at each end, and the shaft has carved, provocative twists. It weighs in at a pound, is more than 9 inches long, and its heaviness and smoothness, plus the twisties, make this a quality sex toy. You definitely deserve it. (Available from *www.search.stockroom.com*.)

---

four people in one bed **is nothing unusual**

12 A study carried out by researchers from the University of Vermont found that 84 percent of people, while having sex, fantasize about having sex with someone other than the person they're having sex with. Eighty-four percent—that's practically everybody! Another survey put the number at only 70 percent, but still.... This means that the average sex act involves four people, even if two are "virtual."

No doubt, many people are dismayed by their own frequent fantasies, perhaps even feeling guilty of what Jimmy Carter once called "committing adultery in my heart," because he imagined having relations with women he wasn't married to. Well, guess what, Jimmy? Rosalind may be ahead of you in that department, because even while entwined physically and emotionally with a loved partner, many, perhaps *most* people, are having sex with someone else. It may be a neighbor, a friend, a sister-in-law, minister Bob, or—frequently—an entirely imaginary person. And the virtual sex is likely to be kinkier than, or at least different, from what's going on in the nonvirtual bed.

The high percentage of other-person fantasies is perhaps proof of the dictum we mentioned early on, about the importance of novelty in stimulating the human brain. Even though we love A, cherish A, and even give A an A+ in sexual relations, there's still that seemingly insatiable desire for novelty—B. As in Bimbo, or Brad Pitt.

You might be wondering if, even though it's commonplace, having mental sex with B somehow degrades a good relationship. On the contrary, another university research project found that *women who fantasized most reported having the best sex lives.*

So fantasy isn't just normal, it's good for you! Some therapists actually recommend dreaming up new fantasies as a valuable method of improving a sexual relationship.

While I have no research to back this up, it seems to me that trying the many variations on sex and romance in this book—which include bringing your fantasies to life—will reduce the need to amuse your libido with psychic stand-ins for your true love.

---

believe it or not #2
come and go at the same time

13 Does it seem like you're always going *somewhere*—to work, Wal-Mart, wherever? Long drives can steal a lot of time that we might rather spend doing more important or enjoyable things—like having orgasms, for instance. Now you can enjoy the latter while still tooling down the highway or caught in a traffic jam. The Auto Vibe Deluxe is a soft-nubbed vibrator that connects with your car's cigarette lighter, has multi-speed controls, and can give you miles of thrills. The vibrator's MPG rating (moans per gallon) hasn't yet received government okay. (Available from *www.lingerietoys.inadult.com*.)

late pregnancy and hot sex: **dangerous or delightful?**

14

Should you happen to be pregnant, I'm sure you already know that sex during a normal, healthy pregnancy, even when you're getting really big, is not considered dangerous. And you've no doubt already discovered that some positions—side-by-side spooning, for instance—are more comfortable than others. But maybe you're still worried that somehow, junior isn't going to appreciate all the excitement and will decide to make an unexpected appearance to see what you two are up to.

Relax. *Really* relax. No less an august body than the National Institute of Environmental Health has determined that having sex—yes, including orgasm—late in pregnancy is not associated with increasing the risk of premature delivery. Actually, it can *decrease* the risk by up to 66 percent! Go figure.

the cat-illac
of sex positions

15 Some years back, a whole book was written about this position, called the CAT, an acronym for coital alignment technique. It was supposedly the greatest sex technique going. I don't think it deserves a whole book, frankly. I'll give it three paragraphs.

Developed by a shrink named Edward Eichel, the position involves the man lying over the woman, and then shifting himself up toward her head so that the base of his penis is held firmly against her clitoris. His body lies on top of her, his arms around her neck. Her legs are wrapped around his with her feet resting on his calves.

From here, they slowly rock on the horizontal, not vertical axis, maintaining full body contact all the while. It's very intimate, very clitoral, and "pushy" on the man's penis. Whether it's the greatest sex position known to man, as its "inventors" claimed, is another story. I'd say it's different enough to be exciting just because it's different. And it may be a little too intimate for some. See what you think.

> TIP: Try turning your head a bit to one side if you feel like you're being smooshed into smotheration.

the **big squeeze**

16

This is really a variation of the missionary position, in which the woman raises her legs, wraps them around the man, and presses her thighs tightly against him, pulling him close.

---

fantasy #3
sex with a leprechaun

17

ST. PATRICK'S DAY

Now that St. Patrick's Day is here, the question inevitably arises in the mind of every woman: What would it be like to have sex with a leprechaun? They *do* have magical powers, you know, and who says those powers do not include Celtic carnality?

To celebrate this holiday as never before, get your man a very handsome Deluxe Leprechaun outfit, complete with velvet collar, lapels, and cuffs; a green vest and green velvet knickers; even shoe buckles. See how magical he really is!

To join him in the spirit of the day, get yourself an Irish step-dancer's outfit, with petticoat, sequin bodice, lace-trimmed blouse, apron, and hat, from *www.anniescostumes.com*. Put on some lively Irish music, pour a couple of Guinnesses, and let the magic happen!

---

is this natural sex pill
for real?

18 All sorts of vitamins, minerals, herbs, and other natural substances have been recommended as enhancers of sexual potency. Probably, 99 percent of these claims are false. In some cases—vitamin C or flaxseed, for instance—the supplement might well improve overall body functioning, and therefore also help the sex function. But whether they have a specific, direct effect on potency is another story.

One possible exception to this general rule might be a supplement called ArginMax. It's composed of L-arginine (which does have a known ability to increase release of the nitric oxide that is necessary for blood-vessel dilation), along with the herbs ginkgo and ginseng (reputed but not proven to help), and a smattering of potentially helpful vitamins and minerals. There is a slightly different formulation for women.

One university study showed that in a group of men (average age, 61) with mild to moderate erectile problems who took ArginMax, 75 percent reported greater sexual satisfaction. Was it just the power of suggestion? Not entirely, because in another group given a look-alike but inactive placebo pill, only 21 percent said the pill helped.

Another study used L-arginine alone, an amino acid sold in health food stores, and found that about one in three men responded well.

There are a great many nonprescription male sexual supplements on the market, but ArginMax seems to be the only one with any kind of placebo-controlled studies behind it. ConsumerLab.com, a pretty serious Web site, calls the evidence in favor of this product "strong." FYI, at the time of this writing, a 3-month supply was about $80 at ArginMax.com, but cheaper at Drugstore.com.

missionary position
upgrade #3

19

This is sweet and simple. The woman brings her knees up to her chest, and places the bottoms of her feet against her partner's chest. Using gentle pressure, she rocks him back and forth, in and out, as she moves her hips up and down. Margo Anand, author of *The Art of Sexual Ecstasy*, remarks on this position that it can "give a sense of power to a man and a sweet taste of surrender to a woman." Wow, that sounds almost better than sex! In any event, it should also get her rocks off because her G-spot gets major action.

ambidextrous
lovemaking

20

Sometimes little changes in routine can make a pleasant difference. Eat on the balcony instead of in the dining room. Broil the fish instead of frying it. Here's a minor change in your foreplay that may provide a minor kick. Every 15, 30, or 60 seconds (vary the times), change from using your dominant hand to your other hand.

For one thing, it'll be coming at him or her from a different direction and angle—one your lover may have never felt before (at least from *you!*) Plus, the nondominant hand is a tad clumsier, slower, more *is-this-the-right way?* That produces a novel sensation (which we know the brain's pleasure centers love), especially when applied to manually pleasuring the most sensitive areas, like the clitoris, or a man's "prostate spot."

---

a special message
for 54-year-old
women

21

Some of you, anyway: Those whose sex drive is still in third gear, and who may feel they are a bit unusual in this regard, especially if their mates seem to have slipped into a lower gear. According to Barbara Keesling, Ph.D., fully two-thirds of middle-age women do not experience *any* decline in libido from what they felt half a lifetime ago. Dr. Keesling suggests the reason may be that as estrogen levels decline with menopause, a woman's testosterone—an important lust hormone—has a relatively greater effect on her. In her book, *Sexual Pleasure*, she cites one study of middle-aged women that found nearly 40 percent complaining they weren't getting enough sex.

So much for the comedian's old line that the foreplay he had with his wife was 30 minutes of begging. Maybe *she* was the one begging!

"Age is something that doesn't matter, unless you are a cheese."
—Billie Burke

> MORAL: **You may need to take more initiative. Hesitant? As we point out elsewhere, couples in which the woman initiates sex as often as the man actually have better sex lives than couples where the man always waves the starting flag.**

zen **sex**

22

"The autumn breeze of a single night of love is better than a hundred thousand years of sterile sitting meditation." —Ikkyu Sojun, revered 15th-century Zen Master

That doesn't imply that Zenful folks have to go through life without feeling the "autumn breeze" of sex. Here, in fact, is a method of lovemaking I learned years ago from Alan Watts, who first popularized this Asian philosophy in the West.

Either he or she lies on the bed, after both have reached a moderate state of arousal. The other person then lies across him or her at a 90-degree angle. (If his head is pointing North, hers is pointing East or West.) He enters her, and they do... *nothing*. No thrusting, pumping, wiggling, or jiggling. No talking. Don't even caress. The point is to concentrate on the experience of being blended with another person, and at just one point—the pubic area. It's all about "Be here now," as Ram Dass put it. Focus your mind on just one thing—what you feel, how you feel, between your legs.

Eventually, if you're wondering, you will begin to get more and more excited. Ideally, you don't move until you reach orgasm, which will be one of the most intense you've ever felt. I found that while this technique has its appeal, I began to run out of patience before long, and felt compelled to throw in some non-Zen moves. Still, I recommend Zen sex not just for its novelty, but because it will allow you, as it does me, to smile slightly and nod knowingly whenever some intellectual mentions Zen-this or Zen-that. 'Cause you did *autumn breeze* Zen!

"feeling playful"
lingerie

23

Certain styles of lingerie are perfect for what might be called a "playful" mood. If you're a man buying a woman lingerie for the first time, and you want to begin on the conservative—but still sexy—side (not a nightgown, for instance), consider a chemise, camisole, or baby doll.

A chemise is essentially a nightgown that got cut off at the top of the thighs, so it's subtly sexy. A camisole is also like a nightie—but one that got cut off around the belly. It's worn with a pair of matching panties or shorts, and shows more than the chemise. The most provocative in the "playful" group is the baby doll, which hangs down to about the hips, and is typically split down the middle. Worn with skimpy panties, the baby doll is frequently made of very sheer fabric, and has a kind of naughty "little girl" look.

the electric **kiss**

24

Whilst engaged in the intimate activity of giving your lover's vagina a hefty dose of oral loving, such as writing her name with the tip of your tongue, try this low-tech, high-touch addition: Hold a vibrator against the side of your writing instrument. The vibrations will be pulsed along your tongue to her, adding new interest to your love story.

dust off that
beanbag chair

25 Beanbag chairs were first in fashion before many of you were even born—which is good, because you might already have one in your attic, or you should be able to get one cheap at a garage sale. If not, they are coming back in style and you can pick one up in many discount and department stores.

Beanbag chairs, you see, are the perfect furniture on which to have a quickie. No athletics involved, no instructions needed: one partner sits *in*, the other *on*. The low munchkin-like profile and enveloping sides make a perfect secret boudoir for an adventure on your balcony or deck.

watching the world's
most romantic movies

26

Romantic movies can often be just as stimulating as "sexy" movies—or even more so. Here are a few that seem to be popular favorites:

Sleepless in Seattle, You've Got Mail, When Harry Met Sally (all starring Meg Ryan!), *An Affair to Remember, Pretty Woman* (my wife's favorites), *Titanic, Love Story, Jerry Maguire, Gone with the Wind, Casablanca, Ghost, City of Angels, Doctor Zhivago, Ice Castles, Eternal Sunshine of the Spotless Mind, Somewhere in Time.*

My own favorites: *An Officer and a Gentleman, Moonstruck,* and *While You Were Sleeping.*

a rose like **no other**

27

This is the most elegant dildo we've seen; elegant enough—even romantic enough—to make a stunning (in more ways than one) gift for that special woman. Formed of high-quality glass, it has a long crystal-like shaft that culminates in a small snow globe, inside of which is a single, frosted red rose. The exterior is exceptionally smooth, and for added pleasure, you can warm it in hot water or chill it, and it'll hold the temperature long enough to be savored.

Because of its high quality and beautiful design, its price is higher than ordinary dildos, but if you want to get something nice enough for, say, a birthday gift, this is a fine choice. (Available from *www.wildinsecret.com*.) **TIP:** Buy her something else, too!

join the bwf
(bedroom wrestling federation)

28 Remember playfully wrestling with your sweetheart when you were a teenager? Remember how horny it made you? If your answer is "No—we boxed," skip this section. But if you ever got a charge out of grappling and groping, you should realize that you can still enjoy amorous wrestling as a particularly stimulating form of foreplay.

Fighting—even play fighting—causes a sharp testosterone spike in both sexes. And because it's not an everyday activity (for most of us, anyway), there's the extra excitement of novelty, a known jump-starter of the brain's pleasure centers.

You might want to begin while you're both wearing, well, *something*. Not your Sunday-go-to-meetin' outfits, but perhaps T-shirts and shorts, underwear, or sweats.

Your wrestling shouldn't just involve holding down hands or shoulders, but should include maximum full-body contact (free-style wrestling as opposed to Greco-Roman). This will get you hot in more ways than one. Even hotter if the woman makes the man say "uncle." Every man secretly wants to be wrestled into sexual submission by a lust-crazed Amazon!

the thighmaster

29 The man is first to "assume the position," his shins under him and feet just past his butt. His legs are spread. The woman then assumes a similar position, but between his legs, with her knees riding up his thighs so that they can join together. The man is supporting himself with his hands on the bed; the woman with her hands on the guy's knees. Now she takes control, using her arms to move any which way she desires, while he complements her movements, moving a little backward, for instance, when she does the same.

> NOTE: **This is not recommended if you have bad or sensitive knees.**

the famous
mint-mouth trick

30 Peppermint breath-fresheners can do more than freshen your mouth; they're also excellent at freshening oral sex. Suck on one for a while and then have at it. Both the penis and clitoris get a peculiar and exciting extra *zing* from the mint. Keep a roll in your bedside drawer.

april fool's day
for her

31 Meg Ryan's fake orgasm in *When Harry Met Sally* is now an iconic episode in modern cinema. Your own sweetheart will be able to do a pretty good imitation with this Orgasm Key Chain. Just touch the red lips on this novelty and it releases what's described as a "shuddering female orgasm." (Available from *www.somethingsexyplanet.com*.)

Another gift with a media tie-in is a set of bodacious false nipples, called Bodyperks. Made instantly famous when worn by the women of *Sex and the City*, these silicone nipples fit into a bra, and look pretty fantastic when worn with a tight top or even swimsuit. Maybe she'll think they're not that much of a joke when she notices all the new admiring stares! (Available from *www.sediva.com*.)

To take her to the next stage of nipplemania, get her a pair of adjustable, nonpiercing nipple strobe lights (*www.nawtythings.com*).

april

april fool's day
for him

1 Invite your man to have sex with a new little gizmo you've bought for him. It's actually a very stretchy, clear silicone sleeve, lined on the inside with teasing nodules. Put some lube on him, slip the sleeve on and rub up and down as he gets hard. Meanwhile, you're holding a small plastic device in your other hand. When he gets good and excited, throw the switch and the device projects a realistic, moaning woman's voice. When he stops laughing, turn the thing off and order him to make you moan better than the machine. (Available from *www.luckysextoys.com.*)

photo fun

2 Men like to take (and watch!) erotic movies, and many women enjoy being photographed. A photo session can be a foreplay kind of thing, but the images produced can be stimulating for months—*or years!*

Video shoots of both of you, from a tripod-mounted camera, aren't the best choice; unless you've rehearsed, you get shots of backs and legs and not much else. When one person carefully photographs the other, with a video or still camera, the results are 25 times better, by my calculations. A few tips:

- Use natural light coming in from windows if at all possible. It's much more interesting than artificial light, unless you have professional equipment. Natural light will bring out erotic details, like hair, nipples, and body contours, while a burst from a flash tends to wash them out.

- Take a series of shots (or a video) of the subject undressing. Men enjoy watching their lover doing a slow strip enormously. Make it teasing, naughty: Pulling at the panties is a *must*.

- Wet bodies are erotic bodies. Take shots of her in the shower, with her body drenched and water streaming off her face, breasts, and tummy.

- To make nipples erect, you can use a fan blowing cool air, manual stimulation, or a simple sex toy called a nipple sucker.

- Bodies look way sexier when glistening. Rub her or him all over with massage oil or baby oil.

- To see some truly great erotic nude photographs, and get inspired, visit *www.Hegri-archives.com*.

Ask your partner exactly what he or she would like to see, and shoot it. You may be surprised at what they want; lingerie shots, costume shots, semen-on-the-face shots, and oh-my-God-I-didn't-know-you-were-filming-me! shots, for instance.

missionary position
upgrade #4

3 It's simple, quick, and effective. Instead of placing her legs off to the sides, she angles them nearly straight down, under and between his legs. The result is a tighter fit into her vagina. And let's face it, a tighter fit is a better fit. Her part of the deal is more action against the clitoris.

a florentine is more
than a cookie

4 It's also a little sex trick that, according to Dr. Alex Comfort, of *The Joy of Sex* fame, helps a man get his rocks off, should he need or desire that. It also feels pretty damn good.

The woman uses one thumb and forefinger at the base of his penis to pull back all the penile skin so that he's tight from bottom to top. That's all there is to it, but you may need a little trial-and-error to achieve the pressure that feels great but doesn't hurt.

ringing that
backdoor bell

5 Notice I said "ringing the bell," not barging in. There are two reasons for that: First, you must go very slowly when entering the tightly sphinctered anus, and second, you don't really have to enter very far at all to get mutual enjoyment. While some couples definitely get off with full penetration, most are happy enough in the "foyer."

The first inch of the backdoor is the anus; after that, there's about 5 to 9 inches of rectum. *Neither area normally stores fecal matter.* However, it is true that you could encounter some residue. As a matter of policy, it's always wise to bathe well with soap and warm water beforehand, cleansing the outer area not only of "matter" but potential smell. If you'd feel more comfortable being even more cautious, you can use a disposable enema kit sold in any drugstore. You can use plain water instead of the mix in the container.

The anus, unlike the vagina, has no natural lubricant, so you must supply some, anointing your fingers, penis, plug, vibrator, or whatever you use with a fairly generous amount. Water-based lubes—the same kind used for vaginal sex—are most often recommended, because they don't quickly break down latex condoms as oil-based lubes will. Some may prefer a silicone lubricant for a slipperier feel.

Also unlike the vagina, the anus does not open itself as sexual heat builds. You have to invite it, encourage it, nudge it to open. For shallow entrance, this can be done in a relatively short time by sliding around the rim, and in just a bit, with your fingers.

I think the best way to "ring the backdoor bell" is to employ what's called a "butt plug." This is a bluntly pointed, smooth, and often flexible thingy that is slowly worked into the anus. Most are pretty thin and short (though some can be very long) and normally slip in easily. Most have a flared base so the plug can't get lost in dark deep space. The base is also a good place to put your thumb, and give a squirmy little massage to the target area.

One advantage of the butt plug as a beginning point is that it's psychologically easier to insert one than it is to insert a real live penis. Remember, we're in anal kindergarten. You might want to leave the plug in place all the time you're having another form of sex, or remove it.

If you want to try inserting the penis, it should be done carefully. In fact, it's best if the man places the head of his penis on her anus, and lets her move down, or back onto it (depending on the position used) in her own sweet time. She may want to straddle him as he lies down, lie in front of him in the side-by-side position, or lean against the bed and let him stand behind her. Be aware that if a man has an orgasm while inside her, his hard thrusting can hurt!

Here's an important caution: Anything that touches the anus, even the perimeter, should never then touch the vagina, as a nasty urinary infection will probably result.

the next best thing
to vulcan
mind-melding

To better connect with your partner, before or after sex, here
is a simple technique often suggested by Eastern-influenced
therapists. *Breathe together*. Breath for breath: in... out...
in... out. The one having trouble connecting—perhaps because he
or she feels distracted, bored, alienated, whatever—is the one who
adapts his or her breathing to the partner's. Do it for a few minutes,
while not thinking about anything, but just experience the feeling of
melding (in at least *one* way) with that other, special person.

---

men who take a
vacuum to bed

No, not a vacuum cleaner. I'm referring to the partial vacuum
that draws blood into a man's penis when he needs to be
pumped by a pump. By squeezing away at a bulb, air is

drawn out of a sleeve thing, and since outside air is blocked from entering the chamber, blood flows in because nature abhors a vacuum and men abhor a limp penis.

The use of these devices surely peaked before the advent of Viagra, Levitra, and Cialis and whatever the new hotdog-helpers might be, but did they actually work? *Do* they work? Can I run out right now to the drugstore and get one?

Hell, yes, say urologists. They work fine, the only trouble being that the erections they produce are dismayingly short-term. That failing can he fixed to some degree by slipping on some kind of band, like a cock ring, after the erection forms, to keep the blood more or less trapped inside. And if you want a really good pump, doctors suggest getting a prescription, because the Rx ones are designed to have a tighter seal at the base of the penis. With a lousy seal, you get a Mickey Mouse erection.

go back to school:
study striptease!

8

In today's fitness world, possibly the hottest trend—in more ways than one—is the *striptease class*. Born only a few years ago, in a Crunch Gym in Los Angeles, when Jeff Costa introduced Cardio Striptease, it caught on like the proverbial wildfire. In just a few years, gyms and clubs across America were offering similar classes.

The line on these classes is that they're lots of fun, actually do teach you to strip erotically, build physical self-confidence, and give you a moderate workout, all at the same time. In some classes, you go through the exercises wearing a feather boa (*and* an exercise outfit)!

If you can't find a class in your area, there are numerous DVDs. Sorting through some details and reviews, I can suggest checking out the following, on Amazon, or elsewhere: *Carmen Electra's Aerobic Striptease, Loving Sex—Erotic Strip Dancing,* and *I Want to Strip for My Man, But I Don't Know How.*

Actress Sheila Kelley (*L.A. Law*) has a book, DVD, and studio all teaching fitness through stripping: see *www.sfactor.com.*

"68"

9 Real 69 is rather awkward and uncomfortable. More technically, each partner's tongue is in the wrong angle for giving the most pleasure—upstrokes from the front being generally more pleasing to both. On the other hand, there is something to be said for the tit-for-tatness of 69, or its shared intimacy, if that sounds better. So here is a variation I call 68.

Let's say the man is performing the honors on his sweetheart. He's all alone down there, poor thing. So she takes his finger in her mouth and sucks it. He'll love that, believe me. Even better, she can use her tongue and lips for what I call sexual instant messaging: If she wants faster, she *does* faster on him...or slower...more tenderly... or more forcefully. He gets the message and obliges.

If she is pleasuring him, her hand may not reach his mouth easily, so he props himself up with pillows to be closer to her. From time to time, he may want to take her finger out and caress the underside with his tongue, or even do a bit of nibbling around her first knuckle, if that's what he'd like on himself. It's a hot technique.

sweeten up a sourpuss
technique #1 diet

10

Scientists at Kaiser-Permanente in Oakland, California, made an astonishing discovery. Studying some 3,600 men and women, they found that eating at least one serving of fatty fish a week gives one a more pleasant personality. On tests, eating fish produced lower scores for anger, hostility, aggression, cynicism, and mistrust. Average lowering was 20 percent, which seems just large enough to make a real difference in how lovable your partner is. Fatty fish include salmon, herring, tuna, and mackerel.

Why in the world would eating fish affect a person's emotions? Well, these fish have high amounts of omega-3 fatty acids, known to be protective to the heart and good for nerves. The investigating scientists theorize that the omega-3 fats give you smoother-functioning brain pathways, which produce a more positive outlook.

If you don't like fish, flaxseed is quite high in omega-3's. Ground flaxseed, which you can buy at health-food stores and some supermarkets, actually tastes quite good sprinkled on cereal. Walnuts are another good nonfish source.

doggy-style
new trick #1

11

Having assumed the position, and captured the man, she slides down until her stomach is smack against the sheet. From this orientation, there is more friction and therefore sensation for both puppies. Some may find that a pillow under her pubic area is helpful.

sex with
office supplies

12

Sometimes you want to do something kind of kinky, but funny-kinky. Here's an idea taking off on the theme of "you're my love slave," where lovers take turns calling all the shots (so to speak). The person whose turn it is to be boss tonight goes to the bedroom, undresses, and affixes any number of Post-it Notes to his or her body. On each note—the 3-by-3-inch size, not the little ones—the person writes instructions as to what is desired: massage... kiss... tongue dance 'til I say stop, whatever. Put the notes anywhere you want.

Through extensive research, I have found Post-it Notes stick very nicely to skin, and just lightly to, okay, pubic hair. If you do this with Post-it Notes you stole from the office, all the more exciting!

---

the stud **workout**

13 Middle-aged guys who were not exercisers were rounded up by doctors at the University of California at San Diego, and put on a somewhat gung-ho program of aerobic exercise, performed every other day. Though the program was not aimed at improving their sex lives, that's what it did. After 9 months, they reported having sex 30 percent more often than before they got fit.

Some people will find that beginning a walking regimen (about 40 minutes a day) will do the trick for them. If you find you need more, look into a fitness center with supervised sweating.

sex for a
steel-drivin' woman

14

Earlier we discussed what I call "John Henry" sex, named for the railroad worker famed for his power in hammering down spikes. But John Henry, according to the old folk tune, had a girlfriend, usually called Polly Anne, and damn if Polly didn't go out one day when John was ill and hammer steel "just like a man."

In this position, Polly Anne can, like John Henry, move straight up and down to her heart's content, but enjoy it a lot more than pounding spikes.

Instead of kneeling on her lover, Polly Anne *squats* over his steel-hard spike and slowly, teasingly, moves up and down. Now, if your legs aren't as strong as Polly's no doubt were, you can help support yourself by placing your hands on your lover's hips or thighs.

You might want to go down real nice and slow and come up fast, or alternate between slow-downs and fast-downs.

And, if it seems like that steel spike needs some adjustment, you can shift back a ways, and support yourself with your hands just over his knees. This puts more pressure on your clitoris, which I imagine Polly Anne enjoyed a heap.

provocative fact #2
if you have to ask for it...
so much the better

15 If you are hesitant to be the one who gets something started, heed this educational bit of data: Researchers at Illinois State University discovered that women who initiate sex as often as the man in their life report having a more satisfying sex life.

XXXperiment!

16 Having your partner show you what she or he likes is one thing, and it's a good thing, a *crucial* thing. But there's a whole other dimension of possible pleasure and satisfaction that may be waiting for both of you—things neither of you have ever tried before. And not necessarily things like wearing Laura Bush and Colin Powell masks.

Start simple. During almost any position, for instance, the man can either manually stimulate her clitoris or not. Or *she* can. With one, two, or three fingers. With or without lubricant. Lubricants with added zap or regular. A vibrator can be used or not, on her, on him, even both at once. Blindfolds... tying down... spanking. Those are just a few examples from XXXperimental Sex 101.

Keep in mind that before you tried Guinness or sashimi or double-shot lattes, you had no idea what you were missing!

"69½"

17

So, you *still* want to do 69? Okay, try it this way, which is better by at least half a point than the traditional method.

Both partners are lying on their sides, 69-style. Each partner then slips a thigh under the other's head to act as a "pillow" for their noggins. The man can improve his access to the woman by slipping his upper arm through the crook of the woman's upper thigh and holding it up. The higher he holds, the wider she is opened.

This description is based on the technique described by Dr. Alex Comfort, but here's another tip. You may be more comfortable if, instead of lying parallel to one another, each partner makes a kind of semi-circle with their body. This is especially helpful if the man is six-foot-six and the woman five-foot-six.

lingerie for the
plus-sexy woman

18 Women of generous proportion (and that's most women) don't have to deny themselves the fun and sexiness of dynamite lingerie. Every bit of it is available in plus sizes, and looks as good as—if not better than—regular sizes. From romantic lace baby dolls and chemises to thongs and panties, body stockings, peek-a-boo bras, and even a leather fishnet baby doll, it's all just a mouse click away. While most lingerie Web sites have plus sizes, there are some that specialize in them.

CHECK OUT:
www.hipsandcurves.com
www.largesizelingerie.com
www.lingerieatlarge.com
www.sheerandsultry.com
www.plusintimates.com

sex is not a
spectator sport

19 Many years ago, Masters and Johnson, who revolutionized modern sexual consciousness, coined the term "spectatoring" to refer to the practice some people have of mentally watching, analyzing, even grading their sexual experience, rather than *experiencing* it.

That is a very helpful thought, though it hasn't achieved wide acceptance, as indicated by the fact that my spell-checker has just informed me that there is no such word as "spectatoring," and that I should have written "spattering" or "sputtering." Frankly, I'm not sure if spattering and sputtering in bed is good or bad, but I do know that spectatoring is a pleasure killer.

Philosopher Alan Watts said people imagine that Zen Buddhism is about peeling potatoes while thinking about eternal verities. No, he said, it's about peeling potatoes and thinking about peeling potatoes. Guru Ram Dass became famous with a three-word recipe for happiness: "Be here now."

When making love, be there with all your mind, heart, and body. Don't hover over the bed like an alien spaceship taking notes on human copulatory activity. If your face is in your lover's groin, let your mind be there. And yes, your soul. Don't analyze, *feel*. And if maybe it doesn't feel all that good, your mind should tell you *only* to try something else, then it should shut the hell up.

shock sex #2
the home depot propostion

20 Your man has been a good boy; a very good boy. With no complaint, he went to the hardware store and returned with 3 gallons of paint a tiny shade darker than the color he used to paint the living room just a week ago. He shaved off the beard that's annoyed you for 2 years. Whatever. So you want to do something special for him, *really* special, that does not involve meatloaf.

Here is one suggestion. When he least expects it, and is in a part of the house where you rarely or never have sex—the kitchen, dining room, even the workshop—and where the floor is uncarpeted wood, tile, even concrete, swoop in on him attired only in panties and one other item: kneepads (Home Depot, about $15).

edison probably
never thought
of this

21

Candles are great for setting the mood, but what if—like a friend of mine—you have a phobia about setting your house on fire? With a dozen candles burning, you may find yourself in bed worrying that a sudden gust of wind coming through the window is going to give you the hottest—and last—sex of your life. Dogs with big wagging tails can also be dangerous should they wander into a candle-strewn boudoir.

A simple alternative is to have a supply of just two or three low-wattage bulbs, and I mean low, like 25- or even 15-watters. This is a secret used by lighting experts who get big bucks for installing that romantic ambience in expensive restaurants. Personally, I enjoy this ambience, until I discover I can't read the damn menu. But since I rarely have to read a menu in bed, no problem. Keep the bulbs in a drawer and replace the 75-watters when you're ready for love.

Plan B: Install a dimmer switch.

missionary position
upgrade #5

22 The woman places both knees flat against the man's chest, which is a way of controlling his movements and tempo. It also makes for a tighter fit. Or, just one knee can be against him, while her other leg is extended to the side. Either way, her hamstrings have to be pretty flexible.

---

the upside of
small boobs

23 Last year, more than 250,000 women in America had surgery to build bigger breasts. Big boobs do have a certain mystique, to be sure. But here's something many people—female and male—don't realize: Large breasts are stunningly less sensitive than small breasts.

This research was not done at Hooters, either, but at the University of Vienna, where doctors found that on average, large breasts were 24 percent less sensitive than small ones. This lack apparently results from the nerves in big boobs being stretched.

What's more, if the breasts are big and droopy, there's even more stretching, and less sensation. Now put the large-breasted woman in the on-top position, with her twin beauties bouncing sexily in front of her lover's mouth, and there's still more stretching going on.

The moral of this story is 1) maybe you should walk, not run, to get a boob job, and 2) if your breasts are already of generous size, you may respond well to a greater degree of stimulation. Which could be fun all around!

double thumbs-up
rouser

24 The thumbs are not used often enough in sex, perhaps because they're simply outnumbered by all those fingers. And remember, opposable thumbs are one of the chief anatomical features that set us off from earlier life forms, so using them creatively celebrates our humanity!

One good way for a woman to employ her strongest digits is to use both of them to massage just under her man's scrotum, an area adjacent to his sensitive prostate. Then her thumbs can move in opposite directions, moving around the sides of his entire unit, applying firm massage with small circular movements. Don't skip the oft-neglected arch that swings over the top of his penis; many men will find this an unexpected treat!

When the man is fully erect, she uses her thumbs to gently massage the undershaft of his penis. A good finishing position is one thumb under his scrotum (again), while the other is making tiny circles in the notch on the south side of his erection.

A man can gainfully employ his thumbs by massaging the area around her clitoris with both at the same time, and then moving one down to rim her bum hole.

walk on the **wild side**

25

Why is it that so many "personal" ads placed in newspapers mention the writer's enjoyment of "long walks on the beach"? Could it be that these writers (mostly women, I think) instinctively know what recent research has revealed to urologists: To wit, that men who walk 2 miles a day have just *half* the erection problems of less-active men?

Probably not. Still, it's fascinating to know that besides the physical, romantic, even spiritual benefits of walking, there's the benefit of better blood flow to a man's dingdorum. Or maybe, all the other stuff is the bonus.

In any event, walking 2 miles will take an average of about 40 minutes, give or take, and you needn't do it all in one session. Think about that 50 percent reduction in problems—it's like getting free, painless surgery!

---

arbor day sex

26

ARBOR DAY (LAST FRIDAY IN APRIL)

Positions and techniques don't always have to "work" to be successful. Many are erotic and fun just in the attempt, and make a good lead-in to another approach that leads you to climax. Here's a good example, from the sex classic, *Kama Sutra*, which the ancient ones, in their ancient way, called "climbing the tree."

The woman stands directly before her man, and teasingly places part of one foot on his foot. Her other leg sort of curls around his opposite thigh. She grips his back with one hand, while the other goes over his shoulder and gets a good grip. Lifting her head toward his eager mouth, she then tries to climb him. Maybe he'll help her by giving her tush a lift. Exactly where and how well you'll connect depends on height difference, and how many trees you shimmied up as a kid.

---

sex with the boss's secretary

27 ADMINISTRATIVE PROFESSIONALS DAY
(LAST WEDNESDAY IN APRIL)

Once I conducted a survey of thousands of thirtysomething-year-old men about sex at work, and made an astonishing discovery. In answer to a question about their most frequent sexual fantasy while at work, more than 80 percent had the same answer, using almost exactly the same words: "Have sex with the boss's secretary—*on his desk*." Quite a few added that this involved "taking her from behind."

To make this fantasy come true, invite your woman to lie

face-down on the edge of the bed, with her hips just over the side, and her feet on the floor. Take hold of her legs, on her lower thighs, spread them, and enter her. A bed is not exactly a big fancy desk, but it's a lot more comfortable for the "secretary," I can guarantee you.

This position allows the man ample freedom for thrusting, which adds to his sense of mastery, while affording his partner intense G-spot stimulation.

Add a realistic touch: She's fully clothed and wearing a tear-away thong.

casual friday **sex**

28

What, exactly, constitutes a sexy outfit for a woman? Usually we think of a slinky low-cut gown or skimpy lingerie. But this all-dolled-up approach isn't the only one that works magic on a man's desire. Sometimes, just the opposite is true.

Men often find an old T-shirt (torn is even better) to be very sexy. And old, faded short shorts that profile the butt are more exciting to many men than expensive jeans that look like they were sprayed on. One survey of men revealed that a woman wearing a baseball cap, with her hair in a ponytail falling through the back of the hat, is exceptionally sexy. White sweat socks also have a peculiar charm. Mentalist Marc Salem says such socks also put the wearer in a better mood. You're "freer, brighter, lighter," he says.

You have to be casual carefully, though. Long hiking shorts, for instance, are not the least bit sexy. T-shirts that look brand new, even pressed, are unexciting. Worse is a race tee that says "Annual Irritable Bowel Run/Walk" and sports the names of 15 race sponsors. Worst of all is wearing those sexy white socks with sandals.

---

get-to-the-point
vibrators

29 Some vibrators are designed to stimulate strategic areas of the vagina. A very popular model is the Hitachi Magic Wand, meant to provide direct, strong vibrations to the clitoris. It's a plug-in, and so has more power than a battery unit, and sports a broad, blunt tip that sends exquisite waves of pleasure to where they're most appreciated. Unlike the rabbit models, these wands are not really designed to be inserted. They don't need to be. If there is anything that could be called a fail-safe orgasm producer, this is it.

There are also vibrators that are curved in such a manner as to provide maximum pleasure to the G-spot. Simply point the curve to the upper, or front, wall of the vagina, and find the exact spot that says "Yes!"

This same shape can be used on him for partial anal insertion in such a way that the curve points towards the man's belly. About 3 inches or so in should do a fantastic job on his prostate.

> **NOTE: No sex toy should be inserted or even placed near the anus and then inserted into the vagina. A bad urinary infection will likely result. Even if all toys are washed in antibacterial soap (recommended!), it's best to keep separate units for anal and vaginal play.**

missionary position
upgrade #6

30

The woman merely folds and crosses her legs so that her knees are resting on her own abdomen. Tightens things up a bit.

may

maypole day **sex**

MAYPOLE DAY

This is not exactly what you'd do if you were circling a maypole in Hyde Park, but it celebrates the same idea—only with *two* maypoles.

The man is comfortably on his back, with his right leg flat and the left bent so that his knee is pointing up. The woman lowers herself onto her excited lover (that's maypole #1) in a sidewise direction facing his raised knee. Holding his knee (that's maypole #2), with her right arm, she slides back and forth, hither and yon, using the leverage of his knee to increase the friction.

And remember, whenever you partner has a leg raised, they deserve something special. In this case, the woman could take two fingertips of her right hand and give him a stirring massage just below his sac when she senses his maypole ready to blossom.

---

the best natural
testosterone pump

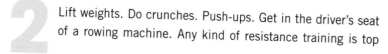

Lift weights. Do crunches. Push-ups. Get in the driver's seat of a rowing machine. Any kind of resistance training is top dog when it comes to boosting a man's testosterone level (aside from taking drugs). A man who grunts in the gym is more likely to grunt in bed tonight than the guy dancing on the elliptical trainer.

Other forms of exercise (tennis, aerobics, swimming, running, etc.) are great in their own ways and can improve a man's sex life by other means—like boosting his circulation. But when it comes to the number-one male sex hormone, nothing works as well as the hard pushing and pulling of resistance training.

To maximize the testosterone boost you get in the gym, use heavier weights with fewer repetitions. Take long enough breaks so that you can do about three sets. And concentrate on lifts that involve *groups* of muscles, like the bench press or slow-motion lunges.

Scientists at Baylor University have taken measurements revealing that testosterone peaks about 48 hours after a good lifting session. Another reason to keep an exercise log!

the lotus seat

3 The woman sits facing her man, opens her knees, and places her legs around him, crossing her calves behind him. The intimate, symmetrical position—he's in the same position—reminded the ancient Indians of the beautiful flower.

give her the
secret sign

4 Even experienced, long-time lovers sometimes wonder if their partner would like sex tonight. If yes, you might want to turn off the TV earlier, skip the last glass of vino, and be sure to clean your teeth of pungent odors and pieces of chicken leg.

A helpful, comfortable way to know what the night is going to bring is to have a secret sign between you and your lover. Hum a few bars from a special tune. Take off all your jewelry and put it down—where he or she is sure to notice. Light a candle. Turn the dimmer down to Dusk in the Black Forest.

You'll be amazed how this corny little trick eases your mind, gets you ready, and creates a cute, endearing intimacy between the two of you.

the ultimate
sexercise

5 If you saw a magazine ad that promised you could boost both your sexual prowess and pleasure by practicing an exercise you could do while waiting in line at Starbucks, you'd assume it was pure B.S. Funny thing is that it wouldn't be; there *is* such an exercise.

They're called Kegels, named for Arnold Kegel, M.D., who popularized them a half-century ago. His patients were women who had problems with urinary incontinence. His treatment consisted of the regular performance of an exercise in which you alternately squeeze and relax pelvic muscles as if you were halting and then releasing the flow of urine. Though these exercises had been developed earlier, Kegel added a simple device that allowed the women to gauge the power of their squeezes—a technique we now call biofeedback.

Kegels proved to be a great way to train yourself to control the urine leakage problem, but something unexpected popped up. Many of the women reported that they were getting sexually aroused more easily, lubricating faster, and having more and better orgasms (some for the first time!).

Skip ahead some years. Doctors had men try the exercises. Results? More intense orgasms and fewer problems with premature ejaculation. Most recently, one study found that 40 percent of impotent men who did Kegels religiously for 6 months regained healthy sexual ability.

All that—for *both* sexes—from a simple exercise? Incredibly, yes!

My guess is that many people try these exercises for a minute or two, get bored, and give up. That's like doing seven push-ups and expecting your chest to sprout bulging pecs. It takes from 3 to 6 weeks of regular practice to see results, which, if you think about it, is just about the same amount of time it takes to see exercise results on your visible muscles.

The simplest way to perform Kegels is to first tighten, then relax the muscles you use to stop urination. Begin with a squeeze that lasts about 3 seconds, followed by the same length of relaxation. Repeat ten times. Do the routine two or three times a day.

After a while, your strength will increase, and you'll be able to do more and more. Eventually, you should be holding each squeeze and each release for 10 seconds each, ten cycles in a row. Repeat the regimen up to ten times a day, which seems like a lot, but remember, you can do these exercises anywhere, anytime.

It will probably help if you use some actual resistance as you exercise. Women can do this by inserting two fingers, spread apart, in their vagina, and using the pelvic floor muscles to push them together. Men need an erection to perform the exercises, which they accomplish by draping a wet washcloth over their penis and lifting up the cloth.

A urologist has developed something called the Gyneflex, a plastic device shaped like a wishbone, which is inserted in the vagina and squeezed. One doctor said this can "revolutionize" a woman's sex life, regardless of age. There is also a more sophisticated device called MySelf Personal Trainer, which supplies not only resistance, but an electronic feedback unit so a woman can see how much pressure she's exerting.

A possible bonus with these exercises is a greater ability to literally grab a man's penis with your vaginal walls when he is inside you, and give both of you a big extra thrill.

charles darwin
oral sex

The impulse to gently bite the object of our passion, and to experience the sensation of being nibbled while in the throes of passion, has a definite animalistic quality to it. Charles Darwin, the father of modern evolutionary theory, thought as much, speculating in his journal that the urge was probably passed down to us from our "distant ancestors."

Earlobes and buns are popular nibbling venues. But they won't respond the way a man's penis will. Yes, you *can* bite a man there, providing you do it correctly. When his penis is fully rigid, and not before then, slip your mouth over it, and as you approach the ridge of the head of his penis, let your teeth make gentle contact with his skin. Pull them just over the flare of the ridge, and stop right there—don't move closer to the tip. Many men will find this incredibly stimulating. It's a good move to make just before you want him to enter you.

provocative fact #3
what women want more of most

7 Ninety percent of women will already know the answer to this, but not nearly as many men do.

A psychologist surveyed a large number of women, asking them, "What is the number-one thing you want more of in your sexual relationship?"

The most common answer was that they want the man to "talk more lovingly." It's interesting that this wish was number one not only among married women, but unmarried as well.

---

sex for gun owners

8 Here's a chance to reap practical benefits from all the time you've spent in the gym building up your guns (or biceps, as normal people call them). Let's assume, first, it's the man who has the golden guns.

His sweetheart is on her back, and he's on his knees, in front of her. He lifts her legs so that they're resting in the crooks of his arms, with her butt raised off the bed. He enters her in this position, and by slightly lifting and lowering her with his chiseled biceps, the man continually changes the sensations both feel.

A woman with really strong arms could do the same, I suppose, but she'd have to be pretty damn strong to hold up her lover's legs and butt.

---

a tip from
martha stewart*

Just before getting into bed, put on sheets and pillowcases fresh and toasty-warm out of the dryer (use scent-free fabric softener). It's so cozy!

*Not THE Martha Stewart; the Martha Stewart from El Paso, Texas, who works the snack bar at Humpty Dan's Bowling Bistro.

striptease **night!**

10

Okay, so you couldn't find one of the striptease classes I mentioned before. You can still do a great strip, though, with a little help.

Music to strip by. Yes, it helps a lot, naturally driving your body into moves that might not be of the everyday kind. After listening to lots of music packaged for stripping, the one album I liked most was the soundtrack to the movie *Striptease*—Joan Jett, Spencer Davis, even Dean Martin—available, along with lots of other stripper music, at *www.amazon.com*.

A sexy costume. Maybe it's just me, but one of the sexiest costumes I've seen is the *I Dream of Jeannie* outfit. It's beautiful, teasing (complete with face veil), and you can get a lot of mileage out of it before you begin peeling away an inch of its sheer blue fabric. A different approach is his-n-her matching stripper costumes—both very skimpy. (Check out these and other costumes at *www.store1.yimg.com*.)

A surprise element. Like pasties! Leather ones, for instance, with tassels—or nipple openings! With matching G-string. (Check out *www.dimout.com*.) We also like Mademoiselle Demure, a set of black-jeweled pasties, black G-string, and "twirlable" pearls, at *www.lingeriegifts.com*. A very big selection is at *www.pastease.com*, including green ones shaped like marijuana leaves!

An extra touch. Two good touches are a big colorful feather boa, for when most or all of your clothes have been tossed, and self-made tear-away garments for dramatically ripping off and tossing at his grinning face!

stand by
your woman

11 I guess an ear, nose, and throat doctor could explain this better, but when a man stands before a woman who is giving him oral sex, the position allows her to take him more fully into her mouth, with less sense of discomfort. And he enjoys much greater freedom of movement. The woman can either sit or kneel on the floor, sit on a chair or a footstool, or lie at the edge of the bed.

Because the man has more power in this position, he must refrain from pushing himself too deeply into her sweet mouth.

---

why cross-dressing is
good for your
sex life

12 There is a natural chemical in a man's perspiration, skin, and hair that has a subtle but definite appeal to a woman, even though she's probably not consciously aware of it. Practical application: To get her in the mood, let her wear your bomber jacket...your scarf...your flannel shirt...or, better yet, your jammies.

The only parallel evidence for men is that they are subconsciously very attracted to the smell of clothing worn by a woman who is ovulating. Then there's the problem of getting him to wear articles of clothing that are pink and three sizes too small.

coming together,
for better or worse

13 Coming together is great, isn't it? Especially since it doesn't happen all that often, it's one of the unexpected goodies that is so exciting to the brain's pleasure centers. But if it never happens to you, take solace in the words of John Gray, Ph.D., author of *Mars and Venus in the Bedroom*. Gray opines that "when a man and woman come together, both individuals are so absorbed with their intense pleasure that in a way the partner is momentarily gone, and the intimacy suddenly disappears."

Gray favors what he calls Polarity Sex, in which the partners take turns focusing their attention on bringing pleasure to the other. So, what do *you* think? Is focusing on bringing your partner to orgasm better than coming together? Discuss at the next DAR meeting.

believe it or not #3
oral sex for narcissistic women

14 Watching yourself have sex in a mirror—cliché though it may be—is a winner. This idea is a little different: a mirror that fits over the man's penis, so she can watch herself close-up (*really* close-up!) giving him oral sex. The 8-inch plastic mirror has a 2-inch hole through which the man's penis and scrotum fit. The bonus is that it keeps annoying pubic hair out of the way! I can't tell you what this is called but you can guess at a visit to *www.secret4us.com*.

the escalator
of love

15

Some 500 years ago a poll was taken in India as to what the most gratifying sexual position was—for both men and women. It wasn't exactly a Harris Poll, but rather an informal poll taken by a gentleman named Shaykh Nefwazi among his friends. Nefwazi described the winning position in his book *The Perfumed Garden*.

The man sits down with his legs stretched out in a Y. The woman then sits down astride his thighs and crosses her legs behind his back. She guides him inside her. "She then places her arms around his neck, and he embraces her sides and waist, and helps her to rise and descend upon him. She must assist in his work."

The assist would evidently result from the woman pressing her heels into the mattress and also using his shoulders for leverage as she moves up and down.

cycling for sex:
the *yes* and the *no*

16

Riding a bike is fun at any age, and if you do ride, you can have more fun later. In Italy, doctors put a group of men who had heart problems on a regimen of regular cycling. In just 2 months, four out of every five said they were having more sex. The docs said biking not only improved blood flow to the penis, but made the men feel better generally, which also helped. So far, so good.

Should you go for a really long bike ride—like the "centuries" or 100-mile road trips serious bikers enjoy—or a whole day's touring across the countryside of some bike-happy place like Italy or France, you have to be careful. At day's end, you could find that you left all your get-up-and-go in the bike's saddle and have none left for your lover's. One study found that *most* avid bikers, even if they don't go in for competition, suffer from some degree of numbness.

It's not simple exhaustion. It's the constant pressure of the bike seat on the tender areas of the groin. You're left numb down there even if the rest of you is feeling fine. And not just men are affected; women can also be left temporarily impaired, say gynecologists.

One measure to take is to be sure you have a saddle wide enough so that your weight is primarily on your butt. Another is to adjust the angle of the saddle so that your weight is not tilted forward, putting the pressure between your legs. It's even a good idea to do this when doing your bike ride in the gym; you'll be more comfortable and last longer.

sex in a
doctor's office

17

Most beds are not high enough for the man to comfortably perform this technique, so you will probably need a table—which tend to be *exactly* the right height—for the woman to lie upon. The trouble with tables is that they're way too hard for anyone to lie on, with one exception: the padded tables you find in doctors' examining rooms. Perhaps you *are* a doctor, in which case, problem solved. If not, you could either slip into a vacant examining room, or boost the height of your bed by piling on a bunch of blankets.

Anyway, this is said to greatly facilitate stimulation of the woman's G-spot, the small area on the front wall of her vagina that's especially sensitive, so it's worth the trouble to find a suitable platform. The technique itself is simple. The woman lies on the bed, tummy up, with her butt at the very edge. He stands before her, and enters her as she places her ankles over his shoulders. Between her hands and her feet, she can guide him into the angles and motions that feel best to her.

stealth **vibrators**

18

Either a woman or her man can handle most of the vibrators mentioned in this book. Some vibrators, though, are clearly designed for a woman to use in a discreet way—a very discreet way. They're not only small but also don't look anything like a vibrator, in case someone should peek inside your purse at an airport security station, for example.

The Incognito from the outside looks like a bottle of pink nail polish remover. Take off the cap, however, and there's a smooth, plastic, multi-speed vibrator. You grasp the "bottle" (which houses three batteries) and massage yourself from any angle. This is a quality vibrator, not a gimmick. (Available from *www.mypleasure.com.*)

Even smaller and more discreet is the Vibrating Lipstick, which has a retractable top like a regular lipstick, only what's underneath is—you guessed it!—a vibrator.

The most discreet of all—it has an *executive* look to it—is the Pen Pal, a combination writing and writhing instrument. The Prussian blue and chrome finish is worthy of boardroom use, while the removable top houses a quiet vibrator. You can even use the vibrator to stop an incipient headache by massaging your temples and the ridges just over your eyebrows—or at least tell a curious friend that's what it's for! (Both of the above available from *www.bettersex.com.*)

let me now
praise your ass

19

"In my sex fantasy, no one loves me for my mind," Nora Ephron once admitted. Nora directed and wrote the screenplay for *You've Got Mail*, so you know she's pretty damn smart. But there's more to even the smartest person than the cerebral cortex and the awards on her shelf.

There's her ass, for instance. Her hips, her breasts, and yes, her tummy. And these parts may need approval, in fact, downright praising, if not actual worship, from her partner.

"Women spend their lives trying to look good for men," says Dr. Helen Fisher bluntly. And the spots many women tend to be most sensitive about aren't their noses or eyebrows, but their rear ends, hips, and waists. And maybe their breasts. These are the areas that need a guy's attention, and not just while he's in the heat of passion. To be believable, he must utter adorations out of the blue, whenever he happens to glance at his beloved. "You have the sweetest ass in the supermarket!" "I love the way those jeans fit you," or "If we weren't in the hotel lobby, I'd pull down your top and make love to those fabulous boobs."

Women will be pleased and assured by such remarks, even if they insist they don't believe them for a minute. Never stop praising her parts.

P.S. You may imagine that the women in question are perhaps too generously endowed in their "sensitive" areas, but even women who are "perfect" (whatever that means) can be seriously lacking in self-ass-steem.

sex for runners

20 This is not yet a track-and-field event, but for anyone who runs and has flexible groin muscles, it will be most enjoyable. She's on top, and slides one knee forward, about a foot or so. Then she slides her other leg back some, resting on her knee or her whole leg, if that feels better. She rides him for a while, then switches legs. The stretched groin area can increase friction and pressure, both in the steady position and while actually switching legs. The man can be on top, too.

head trip #1
the perfect
romantic vacation

21 Real vacations can be very romantic. The best part is that they can be even *more* romantic in recollection than they seemed while you were actually in Yosemite, Cape Cod, or a cruise ship. A kind of warm mist comes over our memory with time, creating a romantic aura that enhances our relationship with whomever we shared the experience.

An alternative approach is to skip the actual vacation and go straight to the romantic aura part. What you do is to sit down over a glass of champagne—or wine that costs at least 9 bucks a bottle—and take turns describing to one another an imaginary vacation that truly represents your idea of the ultimate, absolutely perfect romantic getaway.

"We spent all day on the beach, and snorkeling over the reef, watching beautiful fish of every imaginable color. Then we sat in the hot tub sipping strawberry daiquiris, and now we're at dinner, as the sun is setting. You're wearing a sarong... with nothing under it but lacy panties... hand-woven by brown-skinned virgin maidens. You kick off your sandals... you rub your leg against mine... your foot works its way up higher. And you say to me, 'Tonight we're going to do something we've never done before. Right here in the restaurant.' "

Then it's her turn. Her version might not be so ithyphallic as his, but will reflect what she personally sees as the ultimate romantic getaway.

The purpose is not just to excite or tantalize one another, but to strengthen your bond by sharing intimate desires, under the protective cloak of a fantasy.

'round and around, not up and down

22 Using your hips more like a hula hoop instead of a pile driver is a good and often welcome variation for both men and women. With the woman on top, for instance, instead of going up and down, she can make big or little circles to pleasure both herself and the guy inside the hula hoop. As she swivels frontward, she can lean forward so that her clitoris is rubbing against his pubic bone.

fantasy #5
love your military

ARMED FORCES DAY (3RD SATURDAY IN MAY)

Armed Forces Day, which is somehow different from Memorial Day, is meant to honor the contributions of our nation's military. Nowadays, of course, there are many women in the military, so what better way to show your love for the contemporary fighting force than to have sex with a female boot camp officer?

Or at least, pretend to, with a three-piece costume (top, shorts, hat) from *www.anniescostumes.com*. Add some medals and patches from a military surplus store to make her look so real, you'll obey her every command without question.

Now, boot camp officers are forbidden by Army regulation from wearing a low-cut front with an all-the-way-down zipper, so if that's where you'd like to go, check out the sexy camouflage outfit at *www.electriqueboutique.com*.

instant messaging
during sex

24

A very cool—and very effective—way of telling your lover how you want him or her to do you is what I call instant messaging for sex. It's simpler and even faster than IM on the Internet.

Whatever position you may be in, one lover places their hands on a conveniently reachable part of the other person: shoulders, hips, thighs, wherever. By using squeezes and strokes, the hands-on lover (or squeezer) conveys whether the partner should proceed more slowly, more deeply, go this way or that, back off, whatever. The squeezee instantly obeys the squeezer's every command.

The tongue can also be used to send instant massages. Satisfaction guaranteed, or darn close.

---

one finger
is not enough

25

Slipping one finger into a woman's vagina is what 16-year-old boys do. Real men use three. An old Indian classic sex manual called the *Ananga Ranga* instructs men to use three fingers, all brought together to form what the writer terms an *elephant trunk*. That may sound a bit crude, until you remember that the tip of an elephant's trunk is extremely dexterous and sensitive.

Three fingers are much better at stroking and stimulating all areas of her vagina. Even your thumb can be brought into action on the down stroke, to pleasure her clitoris. And your pinkie—if your hand is big enough—can be gainfully employed stimulating her perineum, the sensitive area just to the rear of her vagina. In fact, you can use both hands at the same time: double-trunk her.

seesaw sex

26

Holding hands is one of the most unusual things people do during sex, but it's a key part of the charm and energy of this position. And, the positions are completely reversible, so long as both have fairly strong arms.

One partner, let's say the woman, lies on her back, with her hips raised, and her legs grasping the sides of the man. The man, inside her, leans forward and extends his hands out over the woman's shoulders. She raises her hands to meet his. They interlock hands. The woman then uses both her hips and arms to seesaw the man back and forth. Then they change places. Playful and passionate at the same time!

---

roadblock remover #3
too much jack = not enough sack

27

We mentioned before that drinking too much before sex is a common cause of poor performance. There's another aspect to drinking that can be even more problematic. Drinking to excess on a steady basis actually causes a hormone shift in men, with testosterone giving way to estrogen. Too much Jack Daniels, in other words, can turn a guy into Jane Daniels. Men who are substantially overweight experience the same hormone change. If a guy is both big *and* a big boozer, he could be really screwed, and his wife not.

It is not my mission here to tell you how to control excessive drinking, but just know that if this is a problem for you, your enjoyment of sex will likely not improve until the boozing is curtailed, either by discipline alone or with the help of a counselor or physician.

butt **beads**

28 Most anal beads are like a pearl necklace not meant to be worn around the neck (unless you're really low on jewelry). Others are more or less embedded on a plastic stick. In either case, the beads are lubed and inserted slowly into the anus. They may feel very good just hanging out there, but some users say the best results are when the beads are withdrawn seconds before climax.

Beads come in various sizes; start small and get bigger if you so desire. Obviously, beads, like all sex toys, but *especially* anal play toys, should be washed with antibacterial soap after each use.

last-second sex tricks
volume I

29 When you *know* your partner is going to climax in a few seconds, there are a number of things you can do to increase the thrill.

Here are just a few:

- Squeeze his nipples.
- When giving oral sex, squeeze your partner's butt. This is easier if the person is standing.
- When the man is just about to climax, use the heel of your hand—if it's free—to push his testicles up toward his body.
- While changing position and technique during sex is a good thing, it's usually a bad thing at the very end. Whatever you're doing, keep it up, and in the same rhythm.
- Barbara Keesling, Ph.D., author of *Sexual Pleasure*, offers a slightly different endgame: When you're a second from climax, stop thrusting and just feel yourself come.

"feeling sexy"
lingerie

30 This is beyond the "playful" look mentioned before, and conveys the message that lust is lapping on the shores of love, that a distant electrical storm is heading your way.

The **teddy**, one of the most popular pieces of lingerie, is shaped like a very sexy one-piece bathing suit, cut so that her thighs and hips are radically bared.

The **teddiette** is the same look, but with garters to hold up long sexy stockings.

The **bustier**, popularized for the modern age by Madonna, is a bra that extends to the waist in a provocative way, and also has garters.

The **corset** is a strapless bustier that shapes the waist, often with laces and hooks for tightening. It barely covers the breasts, which tend to spill over the top. A man may go over the top just looking at this highly erotic classic garment (which Kate Winslet wore in *Titanic*).

The **waist cincher** is a corset that exposes the breasts and has garters. Probably the hottest of the hot!

Build your wardrobe over time. For men, it's the answer to what to buy their woman for her next gift!

sex
in a cage

31 I'm going to present this position in the original words of the *Kama Sutra* (translated from Sanskrit for your convenience) because it's kind of charming as well as being extremely erotic.

"He leans against a wall, and she throws the noose of her arms tightly around his neck and sits in the cage made by his two hands clasped together; she wraps the noose of her thighs around his pelvis in a circle and swings from side to side by shifting from one foot to the other on the wall. This is called 'suspended sex.'"

Wow, one cage, two nooses: It doesn't get much better than that! Seriously, the idea of the woman slowly rotating her body by pressing alternating feet against the wall is, I think, a great moment in sexual physics.

june

why we scream
"oh, god!"

1

"The trouble with being an atheist is that you have no one to talk to during orgasms." —Author unknown

When I read these words, I thought, holy cow, do *other people* do that too? The odd thing is, this habit may involve more than familiar rhetorical patterns.

Recently, neuroscientists discovered that the brain's right prefrontal cortex, where the "orgasm center" is found, is also home to an area whose activity undergoes a righteous spike when we are having spiritual or religious experiences. Does the "Big O" area reach out in its brief moment of neural ecstasy and start talking to the "Big G" area? *Shouting* at it? God only knows.

I am not suggesting for a moment that having an orgasm on Saturday night is a substitute for going to church on Sunday morning. But whether there's a direct neurological connection between these two experiences or not, I think there is some good reason why the temple of love and temple of God are cerebral neighbors.

Many people (you among them?) describe great sex as a "spiritual" experience. That perception is more important than anatomy, in any event, and should encourage all of us to immerse ourselves in its blessings.

breastercourse technique #2
woman on top

2 With this approach, the payload—if you want one at this point—winds up on the man's belly instead on his partner's chin. Belly... chin... chin... belly: If you can't decide, try both, one after the other.

In this version, the man lies back with a pillow or two under his head for a better view. His partner is on her tummy, between his legs, and is high enough up on him so that his penis is between her breasts. If she has to support herself with her forearms, the man can hold her breasts together. He can move himself up and down, or she can slide back and forth on him for the required friction.

This can lead to climax or be enjoyed as a stepping-stone. If he climaxes, the classic curtain call is for one or both partners to rub the ejaculate on his belly, onto her breasts, or both.

"kiss my cinnamon buns!"

3 Here's a great little gift for any occasion—like your Saturday night bath. Philosophy Cinnamon Buns is a fragrant, rich-lathering body wash, shampoo, and conditioner, all in one. Step out of the bath and you're totally edible: cinnamon buns, breasts, feet, the works! (Available at *www.philosophy.com*.)

is the g-spot really in a woman's ears?

4 Most writers on the subject emphasize the need for more verbal communication with a lover. More than 1,500 years ago, the author of the Indian work *Kama Sutra* advised his readers:

"Though a man love a girl ever so much, he never succeeds in winning her without a great deal of talking."

Much more recently, sex therapist Irene Kassorla, Ph.D., stated it even more emphatically:

"Silent lovemaking breeds alienation, increases anxiety, and squelches performance. Talking promotes self-confidence, stimulates action, and increases intimacy."

Author Isabel Allende puts it perhaps more vividly than anyone with her declaration that:

"For women the best aphrodisiacs are words. The G-spot is in the ears."

Put all this together and it seems like a man must begin talking when he first pitches woo to a woman, continue as he arouses her, and keep talking even as he makes love to her. And we haven't even mentioned the need for afterglow chat!

But let's face it: A lot of men aren't that good at talking to women about things of an intimate nature. So what's the solution? Is it, perhaps, the suggestion of legendary baseball player and sage Satchel Paige?

"With women you don't have to talk your head off. You just say a word and let them fill in from there."

When I asked another sage—my wife—how a man can talk to a woman when he has nothing to say, she replied with one word:

"Listen."

Both Satchel and my wife are on the right track, according to a study just completed at the Massachusetts Institute of Technology, of all places. Their conclusion was that to win a woman's heart, it is better for a man to be strong and silent than an oral fire hose.

Yes, you say a few words, as Satchel suggests, but then do as my wife says: listen. As you listen, let her know with your expressions, your body language, and a short question here and there, that you are interested in what she's saying, and want her to keep talking. The woman's reaction to this approach? She will find you nearly irresistible, research declares!

---

give him
reverse oral sex

5 Most often—nearly *always*—a woman begins oral sex at the tip of a man's penis, and works down from there. Try doing the opposite to add an exciting element of novelty to your ministrations.

Approach his penis at the base, from the side, and surround as much of his member as you can with your mouth. From this vantage point, vigorous tongue play is called for. Slowly work your way around the shaft, moving it, or moving yourself so you can cover all latitudes. The bottom side of his penis is apt to be the most sensitive, so dwell there. Then, slowly work your way north. When you finally reach the North Pole, he will be ready to explode every drop of his hot magma.

---

provocative fact #4
beards: the look women can't stand

Men who are trying to connect with a woman—new or familiar—should consider their facial hair as a key part of the package they're offering. Today, there is a strong preference among women for the clean-shaven look, with nearly all considering it a turn-on. If you're trying to connect with a woman who is in her forties, fifties, or beyond, you may not have to shave your muzzy, because older women are more tolerant of facial hair, perhaps a result of growing up with hairy rock stars.

If you want to score, the one beard style to avoid at all costs is the one worn by Dr. C. Everett Koop, erstwhile Surgeon General of the United States: an Amish-style beard, with no moustache to go along with it. A survey found 83 percent of women considered the Koop style repulsive. Composer John Williams often wears the same style beard, but since he's written the film scores to *E.T., Jaws, Star Wars,* and *Raiders of the Lost Ark*, I suppose he could give a damn.

the world's
biggest vibrator

7

It's your washing machine, and the use of this appliance to enhance boffing has become practically folkloric. Either partner can place his or her butt against the machine while it's running, and enjoy vibes that are passed on to the other person as well. If the man is against the machine, he becomes a kind of Maytag vibrator. Have hot water swishing in the machine and adjust the cycles to change vibes. The spin cycle should get you both spinning.

bedside manner,
doggy-style

8 Some people will find it more comfortable and enjoyable to have doggy-style sex if the woman is kneeling at the edge of the bed, and the man standing behind her. Pillows or a bolster can help support her. This way, the man has more freedom and control of his movements than when he is on his knees. She may like it better, too. Some women enjoy supporting themselves in such a way that their nipples are being pushed and pulled on the sheet as the man does his thing.

---

roadblock remover #4
meds and beds

9 If you're suddenly not in the mood all the time or are unable to function normally in bed, consider any medications you're taking. Often, the effect is experienced shortly after beginning a drug, but it may not kick in until later. The important point is that there are tons of meds that can sabotage your love life. Doctors don't always mention this when prescribing them, probably for fear that they're putting an idea into your suggestible little head, or maybe because they don't want to be bothered answering all your questions.

In any event, there are whole long lists of drugs associated with sexual problems, for both men and women. Among blood pressure drugs alone, over a dozen are identified as *frequent* delinquents in this department. Other drugs that are fairly notorious among the docs who keep track of these side effects include pills for cholesterol, allergies, anxiety, depression, and many others—including the motion sickness pills you took before going on that romantic cruise!

Don't just quit taking the medicine, for God's sake. In most cases, there are alternative drugs that are just as effective, but less likely to put a hex on sex. Talk to your doctor. You can do a little research on your own by looking up sexual side effects of drugs on the Web.

---

the kit-and-caboodle
approach

10

It's pretty hard to determine which sex toys are going to be right for you. They can feel different than you imagined, or be bigger, weaker, rougher, or simply less effective than you'd hoped.

The easiest way to avoid disappointment is to purchase one of the numerous kits that virtually all sex-oriented Web sites offer. This strategy has worked for us. If you don't care for one item, simply grab another. These kits tend to be smartly conceived and offer very good value for the money.

A typical example—and one we tried—is called the Deluxe Foreplay To Love Kit, built around a quiet, high-speed vibrator that comes with several attachments, some unusual, good for stimulating breasts and testicles. The vibrator is a plug-in-the-wall model; these are usually the most powerful.

Another kit that looks like a good bet is Toys for Play Kit #1, which has about a dozen components, including a multi-speed vibrator, various sleeves, and insertable balls. If a collection of toys all made of soft jelly sounds interesting, look at the Jr. Bedside Jelly Toy Box. (All kits available from *www.shop.sex-superstore.com*.)

a trick with **a scarf**

11

Silk scarves have many potential uses in lovemaking; this is one you may not have thought of before. I got the idea from Jay Wiseman, who is something of an expert on sex tricks.

Get a silk scarf, not a really good one, but a long one. The woman wraps it loosely around the man's penis and scrotum, and ties a bulky knot on top. Think of this as the bridle. There should be enough scarf free on each side that she can grab hold and gently control him. That's the reins. She pulls him into her, and does what she will. The woman can also try pulling the scarf so that the knot presses against her pleasure button.

Be careful not to give your man *Penis gangrenis*. But he may find that mild pressure from your scarf can help make him harder.

---

shock sex #3
stairway to heaven

12

You want him. He's distracted with one thing or another. You need to really get his attention. This will do it.

While wearing a skirt, remove your panties and continue your normal activities. Somehow, you slyly plan to be going *down* the stairs at the precise moment he's coming *up*. When you're just one step apart, sling one leg over the banister, hike up your skirt, and tell him you want sex right here, right now.

This is a good if unusual position. If he's quite taller than you, the stairs will even out your heights. Kiss him, unbutton your top, make him hot, and you'll soon be on the stairway to heaven!

---

a sweet, sexy mouth

13 Yes, we all know that one's breath should be clean and sweet before initiating even the preliminaries, but many fail to actually *do* something about it. Here are three quick tips that will make your mouth a more inviting orifice to your lover.

Buy an electric toothbrush. Research shows that a good model will clean your mouth 50 percent better than manual brushing. The best choice may be a brush with sonic technology, like Sonicare. The sound waves clean little bits of junk from crevices that other brushes can't reach. One dentist specializing in breath improvement says sonic technology "is the way to go," adding that these brushes will also cause less damaging abrasion than others.

Use a mouthwash after you brush. Mouthwash is a good idea, but many of them have an unpleasant bite. My periodontist recommended a mouthwash called CloSys, which has a unique formulation (chlorine dioxide, if you must know) and has no taste whatsoever. Regular use not only cleans your breath now, but gets rid of plaque that gives you gum problems that produce hard-to-brush-away bad breath. It's available at Walgreen's drugstore and from online sources such as www.dental-mart.com.

Drink green tea. Green tea is very effective at killing the bacteria that cause bad breath. You might want to jazz up the taste with a little honey. New Zealand researchers say that honey (of all things!) not only tends to kill mouth bacteria but also lowers mouth acidity, making the little buggers less likely to cling to your teeth.

the sidewinder

14 Madame lifts her left leg straight up, until it's just about even with the gentleman's right shoulder. Her other leg remains flat on the bed. He then directs his thrusts not in the usual direction, but toward the inner thigh of her leg—the one on the bed. Penetration is tighter for the gentleman and she may be more stimulated as well.

d.i.y. sex builds a
better love shack

15

Masturbation is more common than many people might think. One survey found that one in five women pleasure themselves once a week or so, while numerous surveys reveal that frequent masturbation is practically universal among men.

You might think that all this self-centered activity is among people whose sex lives are pretty miserable, but it turns out that the opposite is true. Every study I've seen has found that people who masturbate pretty often have better and more satisfying sex lives with their partners than people who never go it alone.

This rather odd finding might be simply explained by the fact that people who have enough desire to masturbate also have the requisite desire to have frequent relations. But it could also involve the fact—observed by scientists—that sexual activity of *any* kind increases the levels of hormones, like testosterone, that encourage sex. Fire feeding fire.

Some therapists suggest that masturbation helps people learn how to reach and enjoy climax, and that, in turn, makes them more eager for partner sex. In fact, encouraging masturbation is often the first thing therapists do for clients who are not enjoying good sex. The point is that self-actualized sex does not mean there's anything wrong with your relationship or with you. On the contrary, it's part and parcel of a good sex life.

hot
exercise outfits

16

A sexy workout outfit can be amazingly provocative. Very few women seem to wear one at the gym, which makes them all the sexier when you go for the look. While some can actually be worn to a co-ed gym without causing a major commotion, others would cause every guy in the place to tumble off the treadmill or drop his dumbbells in disbelief. But you can wear a hot outfit around the house, too, whether you have a home gym or not. And, you don't have to be super-fit to look super-sexy in a long bare midriff, with low-cut pants. A nice collection of sexy sportswear can be seen at *www.marimbondo.com*.

---

squiggly-wriggly

17

As the woman is riding on top, she can basically go up and down or round-and-round, or both. But wait a minute: *There are more shapes in geometry than straight lines and circles.* Not to mention the whole world of squiggles!

To facilitate your squiggling and wriggling, you'll find it helps if you place your hands by his sides for better support. One woman likes to make crosses—as in X shapes, not crucifixes, which would be sacrilegious, perhaps. Another favors diamond shapes, at the "bottom" of which pressure on the clitoris is in spades.

Since you can move up and down as well as horizontally, you can even create three-dimensional shapes, like corkscrews, for instance, for an added dimension of fun, if not pleasure.

a low-fat diet
may not be best

Research shows that guys eating a really low-fat diet (one that would have virtually no butter, meat, cheese, oil, etc.) have lower testosterone levels than men who consume slightly more than what the average Joe does.

The thing is, eating a lot of cheeseburgers and pizza isn't good for your sexual health, either. It clogs the arteries that have to bring blood to a man's machinery. If you're on a low-fat regimen, consider adding some good sources of fat to your menu. Any kind of nuts will do, from simple peanuts to macadamias. And instead of eating your salads dry or with some fat-free dressing substitute, use olive oil or a dressing made with canola oil.

---

the here, there, everywhere vibrator

19 The famous "rabbit" vibrator earned its bones by providing deep vaginal penetration and clitoral entertainment at the same time. But you can cover the one missing hot spot with a vibrator that throws anal excitement into the bargain. The top-of-the-line here seems to be the Beyond 2000 Plus unit, which not only vibrates, but rotates and pulsates as well. It has separate controls for the shaft and the clitoral "rabbit," while the anal stimulator is not motorized, and is rather small, designed more for a bit of stimulation than for penetration. (Available at *www.spicygear.net*.)

why men
have nipples

20

So women can kiss them. Lick them. Nibble them. Put whipped cream on them and eat them like little ice cream cones.

Even though a man's nipples may not be as sensitive as a woman's, they are uncharted territory for most men. Few women will have paid any attention to them, much less made love to them in a greedy, lustful manner, as you're going to do. He'll love it.

> **SECRET BONUS: Do unto him exactly as you would have him do unto you. Go ahead and tell him, "That's how I like it, too." You may be amazed at the results when your student reciprocates.**

mystic **sex**

21

Yogi mystics, says Dr. Alex Comfort in *The Joy of Sex*, were deeply into the idea of sex as a form of meditation, even spiritual progression, and recommended being extremely relaxed during congress so as to encourage the proper frame of mind. One position they especially valued is a simple side-by-side technique. The man lies on his left side, the woman on her back, at a right angle to him. She then drapes her legs over his hips, and rests her feet flat on the bed. The man enters her and does his thing as slowly as he can manage. Besides being mystic, it's a good position when you're simply pooped.

the case **for pillows**

22 Placing a pillow under her butt is often recommended for improving the sensation of her pleasure button. The pillow lift also makes for better access to her for both penile and oral sex.

Often it can help when he's on the bottom as well. Another ploy is to place a pillow or two under the man's head while the woman is astride him in an upright position; he can see her better and reach her more easily.

www.liberator.com offers an ingenious series of pillows that zip together or apart and can be used to facilitate just about any sexual position you may care to try. Could be a good investment!

backdoor **kits**

23

As with other varieties of sexual fun, buying a kit made for anal sex is a better place to start than simply buying one thing and hoping you like it. Here's one suggestion: with five anal "probes," as they're called, that vary considerably in shape and size (a good idea!), the Kobe Tai Anal Adventure Kit also includes a vibrator, beads, and a supply of lubricant. (Available from *www.shop.sex-superstore.com*.)

Two other possibilities are the Bottoms Up Kit and Julie Ashton's Anal Beginners Kit. The latter allows you to progress from probes ranging from the still and petite to a King Kong–size vibrator. (Both are available from *www.doc-johnson-sex-toys.com*.)

---

the rickshaw **ride**

24

The man lies on the bed, with his hips and legs over the side. His rickshaw driver backs up to him, and in a standing position, grasps his ankles and backs onto his erect penis. By shimmying back and forth and pumping his legs, she gives both of them a ride to the red light district.

a depressing
dilemma

25 There's nothing more depressing than an antidepressant that makes a man impotent. Yet, a recent study revealed that nearly four out of ten of the millions of men taking such pills experience sexual difficulties as a result. But there are many different medications for depression, and they vary considerably in their effect on a man's sexual vigor. Sometimes taking a Viagra-type stimulant can solve the problem. Talk to your doctor to sort this out; don't just stop taking your medicine!

slap happy

26 A little pat on the skirt-covered tush is to real ass slapping as a regular kiss is to French kissing: The same basic idea made intimate, erotic, even naughty.

Not that we're talking about any level of cruelty here: Ass slapping is a playful thing many men and women enjoy, and it hurts no more than a good massage (and less than one of those killer *deep* massages).

Rubens, most famed for his paintings of buxom, often nude women, was once asked how he knew when to quit working on a piece. "Sir," he replied, "when their backsides look good enough to slap, there's nothing more to do."

Slapping should of course be introduced with the most gentle, affectionate blows. "*Like* that?" If he or she does, you can add a touch more zing. "More?... Harder?"

This can be a good thing just before beginning intercourse.

bring him down
a notch

27

During sex, a man's testes are pulled upward by the automatic reflexive action of certain muscles. That's the same mechanism that pulls his testes in toward his body when he's in cold water, a mechanism believed to help preserve his sperm from getting too chilly. Speculation is that this occurs during sex to keep the family jewels from getting slammed and squashed by, well, *you*.

No problem so far. In fact, from their higher position, his ejaculate has an easier way out. On the other hand, the tightness can be a little uncomfortable for him, and he may appreciate a few gentle tugs to loosen him up.

Gentle tugging during sex can also slow him down some, because his "come" control believes he isn't quite ready for takeoff. This can be used advantageously for both partners.

provocative fact #5
sex and the slob

28 Are you turned off by your man's slovenliness? Perhaps. But it may also turn you on. So say the sex experts at IKEA.

Don't ask me why, but for some reason or other, the furniture chain in 2003 published the results of a survey they took, showing, among other things, that men who jumbled their socks in the drawer had sex three times more per month than guys who neatly folded them. Perhaps the impulsiveness of the jumbler is what gives him the edge in the sex department. Or it may be that he simply has more time available for his wife because he spends so little organizing things. It's a good excuse, anyway!

butterfly
sex

29 By now, just about all the Monarch butterflies will have migrated back to the United States from Mexico, and what better way to celebrate the beauty of their return than to have sex like a butterfly? This position is described in the ancient erotic writings of the Far East, and they thought it resembled the airborne sex of butterflies.

As the man lies on his back, his lover perches directly on top of him. They are aligned at the bottom, because her toes are actually pressing against his. And her hands grasp his, which are held out to the side.

In this orientation, the woman pushes her toes against his to direct her body toward his head, and then slides back again. As the lovers thrill one another, they think butterfly thoughts.

don't nuke **his nooky**

30

You've probably heard of antioxidants. They're natural chemicals found in plant foods that have a remarkably powerful and important role in keeping us healthy. Simply put, they help prevent the process called oxidation, which causes key cells in the body to turn into harmful little gremlins. These gremlins make you old before your time in many different ways and can actually lead to serious disease.

While important for all of us, these antioxidants have a special role to play in protecting a man's sexual function from growing decrepit. With little antioxidant protection, his blood vessels are a lot more likely to become clogged and inflamed, resulting in less and less circulation to his penis.

While nearly all vegetables and fruits have good amounts of these protectors (especially colorful ones like berries, melons, and citrus), the overall champ may well be broccoli. Unfortunately, when broccoli is cooked or reheated in the microwave, virtually all the major antioxidants it packs are nuked into oblivion!

This discovery is quite recent and I well remember that just before I read about it, I'd cooked myself a big mound of broccoli… in the nukerator! No more. All my broccoli is steamed, a process that destroys only a minuscule amount of its health powers.

You can also buy broccoli sprouts in many markets; they're an especially rich source of antioxidants. Put them on any kind of salad or sandwich for a taste and health zing.

july

sex on the beach #1
pitch a tent

It's near the end of a wonderful sun-blasty day. Your partner's warm body is sending you messages. You want to respond. But dare you? On the *beach*?

Yes, you *can* dare. If you're prepared.

First of all, you've waited until the sun is getting ready to call it quits. The great majority of sunbathers have called it quits, too, and headed home with their kids. Preferably, it's near low tide, so the beach is deep, giving you more privacy. You've staked out a spot that is neither too close to the surf, where people might be strolling, nor too close to any boardwalks, decks, or saltwater taffy stores that might happen to be where the sand ends.

Here is what you've brought to the beach with you, besides your sand buckets:

- A large but not too heavy beach umbrella. The one we bought at Wal-Mart cost only about $20, and is over 7 feet wide when fully extended. That's all the room you need.
- A very large beach blanket. Although some people don't mind rolling around bare-ass on sand, others will prefer a blanket.
- A king-size sheet (or two smaller ones).
- A dozen spring-loaded clothespins.
- Optional: two pillows, one for under someone's butt, the other for under the other person's head.

Yes, some assembly is needed, but very little. The umbrella, fully extended, is placed on its side, facing the direction you're most concerned about protecting from busybodies. You might be worried about the umbrella pole, but don't be: Both of you will be able to fit comfortably between the slanting pole closer to the top of the umbrella.

Next, grab the sheet and use the clothespins to fasten it to the rim of the umbrella. Take the other end of the sheet and place it under the sharp tip of the umbrella pole that you usually pitch in the sand, to create yourselves a tent. If it's a little breezy, little piles of sand can be used to hold the sheet from flapping.

Make sure your beach blanket is spread out nice and flat, and that there aren't any seashells underneath it. Put on some music on a boom box to disguise any noises you plan on making and to keep from being spooked by hearing noises made by approaching people (probably imaginary).

Peel off each other's swimsuits—it's best if she wears a bikini that opens from the sides—and enjoy sex on the beach, a pleasure millions dream of but few accomplish!

PLAN B: **Buy a nylon tent.**

ob-gyn sex

2 I have no idea how many people fantasize about being an OB/GYN doc, or having sex with someone who is, but on the chance that there are millions of you, you should know about the Vibrating Pleasure Periscope. This is an all-white medical-looking instrument that can be eased into the body orifice of your choice, and lets you observe what's in there. The rounded clear plastic tip lights up for your viewing pleasure; the vibrator has a separate control. Using both at the same time is bound to result in a blurry image! (Available from *www.extremerestraints.com*.)

---

how to whip up
a sperm storm

3 Part of the excitement of sex for some couples is the promise of creating a baby. If that's the case, it certainly makes sense to send in lots of sperm. Here are two ways to boost not only the quantity, but even the *quality* of sperm.

First, read this book cover-to-cover, because urologists have found that the more aroused a man is when he climaxes, the stronger his muscular contractions, which in turn cause him to ejaculate more sperm, and even "reach back" to get the youngest (and therefore healthier) sperm into the field. Proving this point clinically, some researchers found that when men masturbated while watching X-rated movies, their sperm count was nearly 50 percent higher than when they just wanked off without the extra excitement.

Another technique is for the man to masturbate—but not climax—a few hours before the main event. This is said to get a lot of sperm in the "ready room" and encourage newer, younger sperm to come out as well when the man climaxes.

Fire **works**

4 JULY 4TH (INDEPENDENCE DAY)

One way to add heat to a massage is to simply warm the massage oil in the microwave before use. Always pour it on your hands first—to make sure it's not too cold or too hot.

But if it's hot you want, and the thrill of mild pain, you can enjoy a four- or five-alarm "massage" by dripping candle wax on your lover's thrill-hungry body. You can buy candles specially made so that the wax they produce is not as hot as that from a regular candle.

An intriguing alternative approach is Lava Lotion, a candle that drops wax on the body, but wax that turns into massage oil when it's rubbed in. Always test a candle out first, holding it fairly far away from the skin, and nowhere near the face!

provocative fact #6
suck her penis, in a manner of speaking

Doctors who are experts on embryonic development have found some fascinating things that weren't taught in my freshman biology class. Namely, that the same tissue that in a boy develops into the super-sensitive penis head, develops in the girl child into the nerve-packed clitoris. If a man loves it when his penis head is sucked and licked, he should now know why his sweetheart's clitoris craves and deserves the same treat. And there's more.

The outer vaginal lips of a woman develop out of the same

tissue that in a man winds up as his scrotum. Her inner vaginal lips are the counterpart of the skin on his penis shaft. And some doctors believe that a woman's pleasure-creating G-spot, even though it's not yet considered an "official" organ, is related to a man's prostate, which when pressed from between his legs, or a few inches inside and on the belly side of his anus, greatly stimulates *him*.

"Do unto others as you would have them do unto you" is the most common principle in the world's great religions. Now you know why.

---

a super snack for
on-the-road lovers

Trail mix—a.k.a "gorp"—is a combination of nuts and dried fruits that resists heat, and doesn't get squashed, broken into bits, or become disgustingly soggy, like other portable snacks that you carry in your daypack for hours.

The thing is, nuts and dried fruits all have a very high concentration of just about every nutrient and sexual health-promoting substance known. Here are some of the best choices for your own trail mix recipe:

Walnuts. A leading source of L-arginine, an amino acid that is the precursor of nitric oxide, the key compound your body uses to relax blood vessels and make for better sex (and better circulation). Like other nuts, walnuts are an excellent source of monounsaturated fats, which are powerful boosters of testosterone, and one of the best things in the world for your heart. They also have plenty of fiber, and calories for the energy you need on—and after—long treks.

Almonds. Highest of all nuts in the valuable monos and also unusually high in vitamin E, a powerful antioxidant.

Dried cranberries (as in Craisins). Recently identified as having more antioxidants that keep your circulation flowing smoothly than just about any food in the known universe.

Raisins. Also packed with good stuff for the circulatory system, just like red wine. Raisins are also very rich in the trace mineral boron (as are almonds), believed to be extremely important to a healthy prostate, and scarce in our diet.

Mix these and any other ingredients (I'm partial to dried apricots) and put handfuls in Baggies to carry with you as you roam the world in search of beauty and excitement—and a good place to settle down for a night of love. Your healthy snacks will add power to your passion.

the north-south **move**

7 When she is on top, she moves forward (toward his head) and backward, rather than up and down or in circles. Barbara Keesling, Ph.D., suggests supporting yourself on your elbows, and keeping your butt as high as high as you can (without losing him). Doing this, she says, will maximize contact between his penis and your G-spot. Highly recommended!

---

try the
nipple isolator trick

8 Scientists who measure such things say that the sensitivity of the average woman's nipples and the surrounding areolas is some two to three times *less* than that of her index finger. Well, there are two ways to deal with this fact. One is to make love to her index finger; the other is to use more pressure than you might be used to when stimulating her nipples.

One way to isolate the nipples, which can increase the intensity of the sensation, is to cup her breasts with both hands in such a way that her nipples are protruding from the "V" between any two of your fingers, and focus the attention of your tongue on them. You ought to ask her if you're doing it too hard or not hard enough—or if it feels too weird. Many women like this, though not necessarily for extended periods of time.

---

fantasy #6
be that slut at the office

Coax out of him who he thinks is a hot babe where he works. You're already in the bedroom, and he'll be surprised by your question, but keep after him 'til he coughs up a name.

You *become* her.

You berate his wife or girlfriend (that's *you*) as ordinary and boring. She can't possibly excite him and satisfy him as you will. And you're going to prove it.

You're now a lascivious, no-holds-barred man-stealer.

"Does *she* do this for you?" you demand of him, as you do something you've never done before.

"Can *she* do *this?*" you ask, doing something acrobatic.

Pull out all the stops, so he can fantasize about super-hot sex with the office bitch he named. It'll work out for both of you.

Next time, it's your turn to name a guy you think is hot. Your partner will do everything in his power to match or exceed what *you* did to him!

---

sex in the
swimming pool

Two words: *Bad idea!*

Reason: The chlorine and other chemicals in swimming pools and hot tubs can enter a woman's vagina when she's having intercourse, and cause an irritation that can bother her for a week or more.

Swimming pools are, however, wonderful places for a romantic prelude to sex, in which you can do all sorts of provocative, naughty things, including removing each other's swimsuits (if you had them on to begin with) and watching each other's body parts practically floating. Save the intercourse part for after a shower.

walkin' **the dog**

11 Most often, the man enters the woman doggy-style when she's crouching. But—if varying heights don't interfere—he can also enter her while both are standing. Try this is at the bedroom window—tastefully shrouded by window-box flowers—then slowly walk your way toward the bed, where she can lean over. Or walk anywhere, although I don't suggest walking up and down the stairs.

unsolved mysteries of the sexual universe #1
intimacy

12 What would you imagine your man—or any man—enjoys most about sex?

The sense of conquest? Teasing and being teased? Exploding in orgasm?

Perhaps none of the above. Perhaps it's the... *intimacy*.

A poll of thousands of youngish guys who were asked this question by *Men's Health* magazine, put the answer "conquest" dead last, with only 7 percent saying this was the best part. And listen to this: Only 16 percent put "orgasm" first. "Eroticism" did better at 33 percent, but "intimacy" beat them all, with 44 percent naming it their favorite part of sex!

Maybe the notion that men are all about getting their rocks off is out-of-date, incorrect, or even mythical. In any case, it suggests that giving a man "good loving" may be less mechanistic than we imagine.

Here are some things my men friends and I consider especially "intimate": getting little kisses all around the edges of our mouth; getting kissed on the eyelids, or underarms; being stared at from 6 inches away and told we're incredibly handsome or great lovers; being snuggled up against following sex. One man thought the most "intimate" thing was when, following his climax from oral sex, his wife licked some of his ejaculate from his softening penis.

"bra-vo!"
lingerie

13

Tonight, we feel very sexy, and it's time to wear lingerie that sends that message loud and clear. And what better place to focus our attention than the bra?

The *full-cup* bra covers the breasts completely, but can be made very sexy with a front clasp that either of you can open without warning. The next step is the *half-cup bra*, which exposes the top half of the breasts; a good choice, perhaps, for the woman with fairly generous breasts—very provocative!

Moving right along, we come to the *demi-bra* or *shelf-bra*, which supports the breasts on a "shelf" or underwire demi-cup, leaving the nipples exposed. The bra itself becomes only a symbolic element to help support and highlight the fully exposed breasts. Can there be anything sexier? Possibly. The *open-cup* or *peek-a-boo bra*, which is a regular bra with one small change: holes where the nipples and surrounding skin shine through like the headlights they are.

Can't decide? Get one for every day of the week!

talk up your testosterone

14

Some men may find it hard to have a decent conversation with a woman, but if they do talk, they could be harder later. Scientists from the University of Chicago discovered that when men have just a paltry 5-minute conversation with a woman, their testosterone level, measured 20 minutes post-talk, is 30 percent higher than it was before!

---

watching "how-to" sex videos

15

Not that you *need* to, of course, But *somebody* must, because the ads for Better Sex videos have appeared for a long time in a number of mass-circulation magazines (with very high advertising rates), and they have dozens of titles. So we decided to order a few and take a look-see.

The introductory videos have doctor-type people giving sex advice, and couples demonstrating it. It's sex kindergarten, basically. Watching some of the more advanced videos, the learning curve goes up to third or fourth grade, but maybe higher if you've never enjoyed oral or anal sex.

I finally decided that these videos have a hidden value, in that their clinical approach to all manner of sex play makes it very easy for a couple watching them to discuss what they're seeing. Just like there's usually something on a menu you've never tried before, there will probably be a few things on the more advanced videos that you haven't tasted—at least together. Take a shot at *www.bettersex.com*.

---

fantasy #7
sex with the maid

16

I wonder how many men have been asked by their indignant partner at least once, "Do you think I'm your *maid?*"

Here is a way to answer that irritating question once and for all: a Sexy French Maid outfit! It's like saying, "No, dear, I don't think you're my maid. I just want you to wear this sheer lace baby doll with an open back, tie closures, garters, wristlets, choker, and G-string so you'll *look* like a maid."

If, like so many French maids, she turns out to be ungrateful, you may be forced to buy her a *black vinyl* maid's outfit, with white apron, and one added touch for when she needs to be sternly reminded of her duties—openings for her cheeks. Various options are available from *www.flirtylingerie.com*.

---

blood may be thicker
than water, but...

17 Drinking a couple glasses of water has the unexpected effect of improving blood flow, say scientists, especially to the brain. The brain, you know, the place where the orgasm center is located.

give him
flip-flop tongue

18

Elsewhere, I speak of switching hands when applying various sexual moves, to change the sensation your lover feels. The same idea can be applied to the tongue. Not that you have two tongues, but your tongue has two sides: top and bottom. The topside is relatively smooth; the bottom side more rough and ridgey, as if designed by nature for holding a thermometer in place.

Therefore: after the woman has applied tongue #1 to his hardness, she switches to using tongue #2. A good target area is the bottom side of his penis just behind the head. Switch back and forth; he'll love it.

---

leg men, boob men,
and real men

19

Perception: There are two types of men—the leg man and the boob man.

Reality: These two types of men, between them,

constitute less than 10 percent of all men. Real men, at least statistically average men, much prefer other body parts. In fact, they really aren't "parts" at all.

Men's Health, a magazine forever polling its readers on everything under the sun—and under the sheets—found that the "most important physical trait" a woman can have is...a *pretty face*. Fully 39 percent of their respondents said that. And I might add that their online respondents tend to be young, horny guys. In second place was a sweet smile, and third came a nice butt.

So if your lover thinks you have a pretty face (what *else* would he think?) and if you use it to smile sweetly at him because he's so handsome or helpful or still awake, you've gone a long way toward encouraging him to think you're desirable. Got a nice butt? You're home free! And probably in the bedroom.

beyond stroking—
way beyond

20

Many men will find this the best hand job in the world. Whether offered as a beginning-to-end treat or just one move in a many-splendored love tryst, it provides hard-to-beat direct and strong stimulation. When combined with oral lovemaking, it achieves even higher degrees of ecstasy.

The woman circles the man's penis with her thumb and first finger. If she's right-handed, her left hand goes on first. On top of this ring, she wraps the thumb and first finger of her other, dominant hand. From the base, she moves her hands upward, and as she does so, she twists them in opposite directions. Start slowly, with a loose grip. Move up and down, stopping, in the beginning, just under the head of the penis. As the man becomes increasingly excited, increase first the pressure, then the tempo. Include the head now, as well as the shaft. You may want some lubricant, even if it doesn't seem necessary. Make sure you warm it between your hands before rubbing it on him.

When your hands are at the base of his penis, you can take the rest into your mouth, either all of it, or just the tip. If you're using lubricant, make sure it's the "edible" variety!

If you want him to climax, be sure to have a pillow handy if there's anyone else in the house, because he's going to scream his head off!

This is also a good technique to rouse a man who's already come once, and needs something a little unusual to get him hard again.

the right way **to say something good**

21

The more specific a compliment is, the more believable. When you speak to a lover in the perisexual period (before, during, or after), and you say things like "I love you. You're wonderful. You're sweet. You make me feel good," the other person may well wonder (or even ask you): *why?*

You will have better luck communicating your appreciation by saying things like "You have the most beautiful breasts in the world. Your ass drives me wild. You know just how to get me wet." That's *credibility*.

---

remote-control **sex**

22

You're more or less forced to attend the annual fundraising dinner of the Cement City Art Museum, or some similar event that's not exactly a rave in Knightsbridge. If you want to have some really naughty fun, try remote-control sex.

The idea: a vibrator worn by the woman and controlled remotely by the man. Example: The Remote Control Sea Shell looks like a pink scallop shell and straps around the hips. Made of soft jelly, the shell fits between the legs and has a 2-inch vibrating probe. While she's sitting across the table from him, or chatting it up at the bar, he devilishly turns her on with a three-speed control unit. It has a range of 15 to 20 feet. Besides batteries, you need a good sense of humor! (Available from *www.lingerie.inadult.com.*)

If the idea of warming up your lover while she's in the shower or bath appeals to you, there's a waterproof remote offered at *www.luckysextoys.com.*

sex on the beach #2
for bolder souls

23 Maybe the beach is just about deserted, or maybe you're bolder souls who don't feel compelled to use the beach umbrella and other privacy things described earlier. So, all you need is two large beach blankets, or just one if you get turned on by warm sand on your naked body.

Wrap a blanket completely around both of you, leaving your heads exposed if you want fresh air. Now, the thing is, you may or may not be a tad cautious about letting any other beach visitors notice the motion of your ocean as you're doing it by the sea. For you, I have a special position, in which movement is radically minimized; you could well look like you're hugging, not screwing your brains out.

She lies on her stomach. Her legs are slightly spread, just far enough apart so that he can lie over her, his legs outside hers. He enters her vagina, and as he does so, she draws her legs together, and crosses one ankle over the other.

She's got him trapped tight. So tight he can move only slightly up and down, which is the point of this hideaway position. But the tightness has its rewards in terms of pleasure and intensity. If you're going to have sex on the beach, you might as well go for broke!

---

turn him on
with your afterglow

24

According to the 1,500-year-old advice in the Indian work *Kama Sutra*, "After the intercourse is over, the woman should lie there exhausted with an infatuated expression on her face and close her eyes. This makes a man give his all for her."

bridle 'n' stirrups

25

He's flat on his back and hard as a rock. She lowers herself on to him, with her knees outside his. She then brings her legs together so her feet are hooked over the very bottom of his thighs. That's her stirrups.

Her bridle? It's the ends of the pillow under his head. She grabs them and pulls in rhythm with her hips, which are now raised and free. Alternatively, if she's still a little mad at him for something or other, she can grab hold of his ears.

beyond the belly shirt

26

Looking for something sexy to wear, something beyond the belly shirt look? We've found it for you— in São Paulo, Brazil. Just a day ago, as I'm writing this, a designer at a major fashion show introduced what's been dubbed "Butt Couture." The lovely young model strutting down the runway had on an outfit that was not beachwear, but rather a casual, party look. And about two-thirds of her sexy butt was exposed by the cut of her clothes. No thong, either. Go for it!

the only thing
duct tape
won't do

27 It's not very good for fastening the wrists of a person in mutual bondage. Major drawbacks: can remove a layer or two of epidermal tissue when removed, and leaves a sticky, messy residue on the red marks. This is the conclusion of the author of *Jay Wiseman's Erotic Bondage Handbook*, a man who apparently knows whereof he speaks. After testing various tapes, Wiseman concludes that the best is Scotch Cloth Tape, which is not very sticky and leaves no residue. If you only have, say, adhesive tape, he suggests applying a layer of plastic wrap to the skin, and wrapping the tape over it.

Strips of Velcro can also be used. Or, find a long ribbon and just tie the ends. More comfortable than rope. Just don't make the end knot tight; you'll have to cut it off.

the world's fastest,
cheapest aphrodisiac

28

When I was in high school, I was taught that the difference between humans and all other species was that humans could reason. Then they threw that out and said the one difference was that humans are the only animals that use tools. Soon that, too, went by the wayside. Scientists are still debating this issue.

But I have the answer: Humans are the only animals that wear clothing. *All* of us do. And it's not just a necessity, but a complicated, intensely stylized cultural practice that in many cases amounts to a virtual obsession. Even *Playboy* models and porn stars would never think of going to the mall topless.

Is it any wonder, then, that removing one's clothing in someone else's presence is one of the most provocative acts known?

Back in 1994, a Sex in America survey conducted by researchers at the University of Chicago made this astounding discovery: When a large number of men were queried as to their number-one favorite sexual turn-on, the winner was intercourse. Not surprising. Number three was receiving fellatio. But what was *better* than oral sex? The number-two turn-on was *watching their partner undress.*

Now, these were adult men, not 14-year-old peeping toms watching the girl next door remove her bra. The thrill of watching is both deep-seated and long-lasting, it seems. Particularly with men, who as you already know, are mesmerized by images of naked and near-naked women. The thrill for a woman may be a bit less, but probably not *that* much less.

Doing a striptease for your favorite guy therefore goes to the top of the class as a natural, surefire aphrodisiac. Tease him. Play music, if you like. Start stripping downstairs, perhaps with the famous Janet Jackson ploy. Make him follow you like a dog as you wend your way to the bedroom. You'll be amazed how hot he gets!

it's okay
to be shallow

29 In certain positions, you may well find that male penetration of the vagina is not as deep as you might wish. While deep strokes can be great, the fact is that, during sex, the first 2 inches of the vaginal wall are the most sensitive—and tightest. That, thanks to this area swelling up the most with blood. Shallow thrusting can have a charm all its own.

doin' cats
'n' dogs

30 One of the most basic yoga exercises is getting in an all-fours position, then arching the spine. They call this the "cat" position. Curiously, there is also the "dog" position, in which the spine is dipped down. A combination of these techniques can be nicely employed while having sex doggy-style.

The woman drops down to a position where she's supporting herself on her forearms, while her tush is in the air. She bends her shoulders down and arches her back however much is comfortable. In this position, her vaginal barrel becomes shortened, and the man should feel more friction. Slowly she drops her back and creates a dip, raising her shoulders and head. Now the vagina feels longer, allowing deeper penetration and creating a new sensation for both the man and the woman.

The rhythmic change from up to down will give the head of his penis a great roller-coaster ride!

a rose
to tickle her fancy

31

A classy but sassy gift! This beautiful 20-inch long-stem rose looks like, well, a rose, pretty enough to display and enjoy anywhere in your house. The difference is that the petals are actually feathers. For fiendish tickling. Add a new floral element to foreplay, or elegance to restraint: Tie her up and take out—oh, no—*the rose!* (Available from *www.stockroom.com*.)

august

the real
love potion no. 9

1 Not the one in the classic song composed by Leiber and Stoller; the one I'm talking about was composed by Mother Nature. I call it Love Potion No. 9 because, well, it's a hormone comprised of nine amino acids, but more important, it has a very important effect on our desire to connect deeply with another person.

Its name is oxytocin, and it's best known for two things: helping to expel a baby from the womb when it's time, and strongly encouraging the all-important emotional bonding between mother and child. Recent research, though, has suggested its effects are far broader. In fact, if there is any natural body chemical that could conceivably be called a love potion, it's oxytocin. What's more, there are several ways to increase its activity.

By "love potion," I mean love—*a strong feeling of attachment*—not sex. While testosterone is the best-known sexual hormone, oxytocin is what makes us couples instead of just copulators.

It's worth noting that every mammal on earth has this same hormone, according to Kerstin Uvnäs Moberg, M.D., Ph.D., author of *The Oxytocin Factor*. Besides creating a bond between mother and baby, rising oxytocin levels cause lab animals to have lower blood pressure and pulse rate, feel less stressed, and *become more curious and interested in one another*.

In humans, she points out, lovemaking causes oxytocin levels to rise, while "orgasm releases a flood of oxytocin into the bloodstream." This could be why, the doctor suggests, what begins as a purely sexual relationship often becomes—for better or worse!—a love relationship.

Because sex and bonding go together like, well, love and marriage, it's worth knowing how we can get more oxytocin activity going. One good way is massage. It should be slow, rhythmic massage, and music and candlelight can make the effect greater. What's more, if massage is given on a regular basis, oxytocin goes all the higher. Exercise, especially if it involves a lot of body movement, also raises your love potion levels. Curiously, so does wine. But only in moderate amounts; get bombed and your oxytocin goes into a tailspin.

Daniel Amen, M.D., who calls oxytocin "your brain's love juice," also points out that oxytocin has a sleep-inducing quality, and since a man's levels can rise as much as 500 percent during orgasm, it can literally knock him out. Anthropologists might add that this is all according to plan, because a man who sleeps with the woman he makes love to is apt to become more attached to her.

the **wrench position**

2 There are numerous positions mentioned in this book for creating a tighter fit: This is one of the best.

Lying on her back, she points her legs skyward, bringing them almost, but not quite, together. He kneels before her, gathers her gams, and shifts a little to one side, placing her calves more or less against his chest or over one shoulder. He then leans forward, gets support he may need with his hands on the bed, and does his thing. She feels free to adjust her legs as lust may desire.

---

give her **some balls**

3 One of the most common sex toys, which some women *adore*, are duotone balls that fit into the vagina. The good ones are somewhat over an inch in diameter, and contain metal ball bearings, which roll around and cause very titillating sensations. You can retrieve the balls by tugging on a cord they're connected to. These can be used as a kind of foreplay or worn around the house when you feel so inclined.

A promising pair of balls at a good price, called Futurotic Weighted Balls, is offered at *www.nawtythings.com*. An electronically powered pair that you can command to perform any of 30 different tricks (called Impulse Orgasm Balls Textured) is offered at *www.wylde.com. Play ball!*

---

sweat together;
sweat more later

4 Participating in competitive athletics jacks up men's testosterone, at least over the short term. But when women do the same thing, their testosterone spikes up more than three times as much, hitting 50 percent higher than baseline. Testosterone is not usually thought of as an important female hormone, but it is, for a variety of reasons, and one of them happens to be that as her testosterone spikes, so does her desire to have sex.

Turning out to be a winner (in anything, including business) is a known testosterone booster, too. Which leads to the conclusion that if the woman *wins* the game she's playing, it should help her even more. The best strategy would be for each partner to play on the same team, so both can win, and one doesn't get secretly pissed over having been beaten by the other. Games like volleyball, badminton, doubles tennis, or even something weird like orienteering (where you dash around the countryside with your partner, trying to beat another team's time) are all good choices. Begin your lovemaking in the shower.

shock sex #4
pretty woman

5 Remember the scene in *Pretty Woman* where Richard Gere returns to his suite to discover Julia Roberts waiting for him, and wearing nothing but one of his ties? How could you *forget* it?

I looked at the original screenplay and found that the scene hadn't been written quite this way. What she was supposed to be wearing was some very sexy lingerie. The director evidently understood the power of "shock sex" and changed the scene. My kind of guy!

If your man's taste in ties is so bad that you don't want to wear one to greet him when he comes home, you can buy a small, classy rhinestone tie at *www.wickedtemptations.com*.

---

tongues **with torque**

6 *Eureka!* A vibrator with the shape and feel of a tongue! There are times, after all, when a real tongue grows weary, or its owner goes A.W.O.L. The Mini-Tongue is made with a natural-feeling artificial skin, fashioned into a 5-inch-long tongue that is said to have the shape and texture of a real one. It "flickers and licks" at three speeds, no less. Lube this baby up before turning it loose. Bonus: There's a vibrating "bullet" you can attach to the base for added entertainment. (Available from *www.bettersex.com.*)

Another unit, with less tongue and more vibrator, is the Clit Kisser. Covered with a soft jelly, this is said to be a "best-seller" at *www.xandria.com.* A user's review reveals an unsuspected and momentous alternative application: "Hubby got a surprise when I lubed it up and used it on his ass!"

---

god **and vibrators**

Are you concerned—even perplexed—about how all this sex stuff jibes with the principles given us by the Almighty? Have you wondered, for instance, what the *Holy Bible* has to say about oral sex? Vibrators, edible body paint, and all the rest?

These are not trivial concerns for millions of us, and if you are among them, you should visit the Web site *www.themarriagebed.com.* Operated by Paul and Lori Byerly, both ordained nondenominational ministers, the site is described as "Sex and Intimacy for Married

Christians." It has top-notch, clear information on many sexual subjects, each of which is viewed from the scientific or medical point of view as well as the biblical. An excellent discussion of the G-spot, for instance, includes the opinion that "the G-spot should be seen as one more way God gave us to share in the pleasure of sex." They even declare that "Many scholars of the Song of Solomon are convinced that several passages describe oral sex being performed on both the man and woman." (Check out SS 2:3, 4:16, and 8:2 to see if you agree.)

There's also a lengthy treatise on what they feel is either permitted or forbidden by Scripture.

They even have some links to Christian-oriented shopping sites that sell all sorts of romantic and sexual aids, without any nudity or links to porn sites. I checked out two: *www.books22.com* and *www.mybelovedsgarden.com*. The former is a bit tamer than the latter, though it does offer things like "turbo jelly eggs." The second has a more eclectic selection, including, for instance, edible undies.

grape **aid**

8

Take a bunch of seedless grapes and put them in the freezer for about 15 minutes so they become chilled and a little hard. Take them to the bedroom. Not exactly to eat.

Pick a grape and hold it between your teeth. Tickle her breasts with it. Her nipples. Her belly button. Finally, her sex button.

Either she'll love it or hate it. If she hates it, eat the damn grapes. But the sensation of cold can create very interesting nervous sensations, more than touching her nipples, for example, can. Stick a finger into a bucket of ice cubes and you'll feel the cold all through your hand. That's the idea of grape aid.

---

the missionary position
gone mad

9

The man is over the woman, as they use the missionary position or a slight variation thereof. Then, without withdrawing (if he's able!), he rotates his entire body so that he's now facing her feet. This will create a whole new sensation for both partners. After a bit, the man can rotate himself again. This technique is known as "the windmill," and can only be performed with practice, as you no doubt have already realized.

"did you **come?**"

Every night, millions of men across the globe ask their women this question. I don't have to explain why. But it may not be the best thing to say.

Some women say it *is*. If they haven't climaxed, they want some quick help getting there. And it's better if the man asks her, instead of her having to tell her sex-blasted lover, "Excuse me, but *I* didn't come."

Many other women find the question boorish, even demeaning. It suggests that she didn't show enough excitement to convince her lover that she came. And if, in fact, she didn't, the question seems like a negative on a negative: Not only did she not climax but also now has to make some kind of excuse, give an accounting of her "failure."

Maybe it's not the thought so much as the wording. Phrase it so that there is no implication of noncompliance. "Want more? Can I go down on you? Want some hand jive?" Something along those lines may sound better—especially if you've asked her if she came a hundred times in the last year.

an easy **rope trick**

11 If you want to experiment to see how a little bit of rope bondage feels, this is a very simple technique. One person lies on his or her back and draws up their legs so their thighs are against their lower legs. The other person slings a length of rope around the left thigh, loops it around the lower part of the leg, then goes back and ties the rope over the top of the thigh. Then the right thigh.

Needless to say, the knots should be loose, with just enough pressure to help the person keep their legs bent and close together. A simple, easily untied square knot is best. There should be no pain at all, and no cutting off of circulation. (If there are *any* circulatory problems, forget this.)

The bound person can lie flat on their back, and their legs can be easily spread without discomfort. With help, they can also assume a kneeling position. *Jay Wiseman's Erotic Bondage Handbook*, where I saw this, also suggests the bound person lie on their side or stomach. Always make sure the person is comfortable, and has no trouble breathing. And don't leave the ropes in place for more than a few minutes, in any case.

Two more cautions: Besides what I've already mentioned, you must ask, what if the person *not* bound should for some reason pass out? The other person should be able to wriggle out of whatever they're bound with in no more than seconds.

Sometimes a mutual bondage fantasy scene will involve one person pleading with the other person, "Don't do that!"—of course, not meaning it. Lest there be any confusion, there should be a pre-arranged "escape" word, which means "I want out, *right now!*" It should be a word you wouldn't ordinarily use during your sex play: e.g., "Microsoft!"

don't let him
drink you
under the table

12

Women usually get drunk more easily than men, and the reason is not just their lesser average size. Because a man's body has relatively more muscle than a woman's, he also has a lot more water in his system. When he drinks, this water helps to dilute the booze. She gets no such protection. If the two drink glass for glass (and she's petite while he's light-heavyweight), it's like he's imbibing 80-proof Dewar's while she's knocking back barrel-strength 120-proof Glenfarclas.

In other words, if she keeps up with him at the bar, she may not be able to keep up with him in bed. Because it's hard to keep up when you're asleep.

Besides limiting her drinking to less than his, a woman can also muffle the knockout effect of alcohol by eating something with it. Raw veggies won't do the trick, either. It should be something that has a good amount of both protein and fat. Rack of lamb will do fine, thank you, but so will a burger.

---

ladies and gentlemen,
be seated

13 Do you have an armless chair? If so, great; you can enjoy many variations of comfortable, seated sex. But a chaired arm can also be used for certain configurations.

On an armless chair, the man can sit down and his lover straddles his legs, facing him. They embrace; the woman assumes most control. Helpful when she's pregnant.

She can sit on the man's lap, facing away from him, and control the rhythm with her feet and toes. She should be able to do this even if the chair has arms.

The man can lean back a bit and have his lover sit across him sideways. Interesting and different, and allows the man easy access for manual stimulation of her clitoris.

Athletic variation: This is the seated version of hanging from the chandelier, only upside-down. The woman faces the man on his lap, and then slowly leans back. Under her head and shoulders is either an ottoman or several pillows to support her. She must be careful not to bend his penis down too much (that can do him serious damage when erect). It will provide maximum pressure on the front of her vagina, home base of the G-spot.

is sex animalistic
or highly cerebral?

I used to naively think that sex probably involved just one or two areas of the brain, those that controlled the most primitive, basic functions, like eating and sleeping. Turns out I was way off base. Thanks to the relatively new science of functional MRI, scientists can now pinpoint specific areas of the brain that become more or less active during specific activities.

Helen Fisher, Ph.D., reviews some of this research in her book *Why We Love*, and mentions scads of brain areas now known to get hot and bothered during sexual arousal. The names of these areas aren't particularly romantic, either: it's hard to imagine even the most gifted songwriter penning lyrics along the lines of "C'mon baby, let me light your bilateral cingulate gyrus... your right amygdala... and oh, your ventral striatum!"

To me, this underlines the fact that lovemaking is, without doubt, a highly cerebral activity, perhaps involving even more brain activity and networking between brain areas than reading a book on astrophysics by Stephen Hawking (especially when you can't understand 80 percent of what he's saying!). And that's why so many different things are important in good sex, whether it's candles and lingerie, pleasant fragrances, novelty, fantasy, or words, words, and more words. Not to mention what you had for dinner and worrying if you forgot to re-cork that expensive bottle of pinot noir!

Dr. Fisher even suggests that now that some psychologists claim there should be separate IQs for things like musical ability and leadership, there ought to be a sexual IQ as well. The better you are, including pleasing your partner while pleasing yourself as well, the higher it is.

In all modesty, I therefore suggest that this book could be said to help you increase your IQ—one of them, anyway—by a good 20 to 30 points. Who knows, it could make you a genius!

up tight,
outta sight

15 Doing Kegels—with or without a mechanical helper—is a great way to increase muscle tone and control of the sex muscles. A woman who is a bit loose where she's better off tight might want to try Oh So Tight, an alum-based cream that produces safe, temporary shrinkage when applied to the vaginal walls about an hour before sex. Said to be tasteless and odorless, it has great user reviews at *www.xandria.com*, one of the most reputable erotic gear Web sites.

Fantasy #8
look like
another woman

16 Both men and woman are chronic fantasizers when it comes to sex, and a nearly universal fantasy is having sex with not-the-person-you're-in-bed-with. The fastest way to turn this mental fantasy into a "real" fantasy is to wear a wig. Unfortunately, wigs for men are pretty hard to find, so forget about a Brad Pitt or Denzel Washington look; wigs are for her, even if their effect is mostly for him.

Want to be a redhead with long locks that just cover your breasts? Want a rock-and-roll or punk look? Want to look like that slut at work? Go for it! Your man's brain is always on the prowl for *something* new in the sex area, so looking like someone you're not is guaranteed to be hot. Start looking for a turn-on wig at *www.electriqueboutique.com*.

sex on the beach #3
moonlight sonata

17 If our first two versions of sex on the beach were both a bit too restrained for you, you can dispense with all precautions and restrictions on your motions. Simply wait till there's a full moon, and go to the beach at midnight. Spread a blanket, slowly peel off one another's clothes, and enjoy wild sex to the rhythm of the surf.

Try to come just as a wave crashes. You'll never look at the ocean again without remembering that!

Afterwards, be sure to enjoy the great opportunity for afterglow by moonlight!

doggy-style
new trick #2

18

In most versions of doggy-style, the man is in the superior position. For a different approach to rear entry, the man lies on his back and draws up his knees so they're resting on his chest. The woman sits down on his penis, facing toward where his legs would be if they weren't under his chin, and becomes top dog.

don't talk
when you can grunt

19

I love this advice from John Gray, Ph.D., in his book *Mars and Venus in the Bedroom*. "To give feedback in sex," he writes, "it is best for women to make little noises and not use complete sentences." Complete sentences can be a turn-off because, as he puts it, it's a "subtle clue that she is still in her head and not fully in her body."

Sometimes the clue is not that subtle. Even though it's phrased in a positive way (which I suggest elsewhere), when a lover says, "I'd appreciate it enormously if you would remove your hand from my breast and utilize it in my pubic area," it's sudden death.

Although it's true that men rarely talk in "complete sentences" at *any* time, Dr. Gray does allow them sentence-speak providing the message is concise, as in "I love your breasts!" Perhaps there is no danger of a woman ever thinking a man is "in his head" and in his bed at the same time.

an anal sex trick
(from a guy who should know)

20 To make entry easier and more comfortable, try this. The woman leans over a bed in such a way that she's supporting herself on her chest and tummy, not just with her arms. Her legs, more or less dangling, just make light contact with the floor. Nearly all her weight is on the bed. In this configuration, there is less stress and strain on her when the man enters.

This technique, needless to say, will not work if she's leaning, say, on the TV or sink: much too hard, much too small.

I am not telling you where I got this tip.

Oh, you *insist* on knowing? Very well. I adapted it from advice given by a doctor on how to be more comfortable when undergoing a (sorry!) digital rectal exam.

champagne tastes
and your sex budget

21 You already know that more than one, maybe two drinks an hour can easily dematerialize a man's erection. But did you know that—no matter how romantic it seems—drinking champagne will take the pop out of your cork even faster? It's those little bubbles. Seems they whoosh the alcohol into your system faster than nonbubbly drinks. And the faster the alcohol hits your brain, the faster you get bombed.

'Course, beer has bubbles, too, but Dom Perignon has three times the alcohol per sip as Dom Bud.

Yes, champagne *is* romantic for many folks, but drink it slowly if you plan on having high-proof sex when the bottle's emptied.

---

samantha jones **sex**

22 Kim Cattrall, who did such a great job portraying the ultra-sensual Samantha Jones in *Sex and the City*, recommends this little trick in *Satisfaction: The Art of Female Orgasm,* a book she wrote with her (now-ex) husband.

After sufficiently arousing her, the man slips two fingers deeply enough into her vagina so that they are under her clitoris. Curling his fingers, he pushes up lightly—*one finger a time*—and takes her clitoris in his mouth for sucking and tongue play.

I think I missed that episode.

---

this x **gets an a**

23

This position was popularized by Dr. Alex Comfort in *The Joy of Sex*, who called it "a winner for prolonged slow intercourse." The woman and man are seated facing each other. Both have their legs forward; hers are over his. (Hence the term "X" position.) They join. They clasp hands. Slowly, each drifts backward until they are flat on their backs, still holding hands.

There can be tremendous tension both on the man's penis and the woman's G-spot as his penis naturally tries to spring up. "Slow, coordinated wriggling motions" are what Dr. Comfort calls for here, not any sort of thrusting, bouncing, or bopping.

If you are uncomfortable in this position, you can periodically modify it by releasing your hand clasp, rising up a bit, and supporting yourself on your elbows. Yes, it's definitely a winner!

bungee humping

24 Sex under partial weightlessness can be fun for some and even better for others who may have difficulty assuming certain positions. When you're suspended from the ceiling by a bungee cord with your body in a harness system, there's a strange lightness and freedom that can prove most erotic. Not to mention the novelty of it all, a quality we know the brain's pleasure centers hanker for! (Available from *www.1sn.com.*)

---

mouth **music**

25 Stick a finger in your mouth. Notice the sensation. Now start humming, using long, deep notes. Feel the subtle vibrations in your finger?

Try humming when you're giving oral sex. Though the tongue can transmit the hum-thrum to your partner, it works best if your lips are firmly against their tender parts, as they will be when you're sucking her vagina or clitoris, or your mouth and tongue are engaged with his penis. The vibes are subtle, yes, but intimate.

A fancy variation of basic humming involves rubbing some lubricant on a man's scrotum, encasing it with plastic wrap, and putting your mouth against the wrap while humming. You can either hum random notes, or an actual tune. Maybe your partner will even hum along with you!

one leg up,
one leg down

26

The woman, on her back, places one leg over her lover's shoulder, and with his help, extends her other leg flat against the bed and out to the side a bit. Or, if the shoulder gambit is awkward, she simply points that leg toward the ceiling. Every minute or so, switch legs. Better than flatlander sex.

the landing strip
on her areola

27 According to one medical researcher, the most sensitive part of a woman's areola—the circle surrounding her nipple—is mostly above it, inside an arc between the 10 o'clock and 2 o'clock. Further, the areola actually has more excitement receptors than the nipple, so be advised: By "overshooting" the apparent pleasure center, your tongue will be landing on a better target.

---

the one reason to go
to a nude beach

28 Maybe I'm a bit of a prude, or just boringly normal, but going to a totally nude beach has never appealed to me (except when I was 13).

Everyone knows it's important to put on plenty of sunscreen with a high SPF when you visit the beach, and obviously, if you're totally nude, you need protection in places where you've never needed it before. Specifically, your penis. Unless you want it looking like a well-done hot dog by 3:00 P.M., you have to coat that raw frank, and the rest of your body, with lotion. Everyone knows that this is best done by someone else, in this case, your beach companion.

Have her begin with your shoulders and neck, and work down to your chest, belly, back, and legs. Then comes the most important part—the application to your willy. This must be done slowly, thoughtfully, lovingly. And don't forget the scrotum! Compliment her on the good job she's doing, the artful use of her hands, wrist, and fingers.

Soon you'll be ready to head out onto the beach, a well-protected, happy man, who doesn't have to worry about getting an embarrassing erection...for at least 20 minutes or so.

the monkey as
organ grinder

29

The ancient Eastern sexual sages had a penchant for naming every position after some animal. One in particular is called the monkey position, because the woman hangs onto and plays with her lover, as though she were a monkey.

The man is seated, and she's seated over his loins, her legs grasping his sides. Though she can monkey around into any position, it will help if she leans back a bit and places one hand on his leg for leverage in her monkey movements. Her other hand can grasp his hair and pull it this way and that, or if his hair is too short to hold, she can grab his coconut head and use that for leverage.

She should *definitely* make monkey noises!

give him a
nipple massage

30

Not *his* nipples: *yours*. He's on his stomach, and you're hovering over him like a masseuse—a naughty masseuse. With your hands at his sides, supporting you, slowly and artfully let your nipples "massage" his back. You might start with his calves, work up to behind the knees, the buttocks, back, and neck. You may find this stimulating yourself if your nipples like the sensation of touring his body. If it's irritating, the hell with it.

When your tour is complete, turn him over by gently grabbing his hair, and massage his front. You might want to use some light lube or massage oil.

A super-hot tease!

---

ringy-dingy **sex**

31 Doctors would say that the best type of cock ring—a device that fastens around the penis to prevent the escape of blood, thereby hardening and prolonging an erection—is the fully adjustable kind. The idea is not to have the thing clasp a man too hard.

But many men like to at least experiment with something that's not only a ring, but has an added ding for the woman. Usually, these rings are made of a soft, jellylike plastic that is stretchable so that one size (theoretically) fits all.

A cute example is the ClitBuddy Buzzy Bear. This consists of a soft jelly ring to encircle the penis, topped with a little baby bear that can be rubbed against the woman. The bear is given considerable help by a small wireless vibrator, whose buzz can be felt by both lovers.

Another interesting him-and-her pleaser that gets a little into the rubber look is the black latex Adonis Pouch Stimulator. This baby fits not only around the base of the penis shaft but also the scrotum. Just under the scrotum, there's a vibrator that sends sensations right through the man into the woman.

Let's see, we're hardening the penis, buzzing the clitoris, vibrating the balls. Did we leave anything out? Ah, yes, there's at least one cock ring that's designed to provide anal entertainment along with male engorgement. It consists of a soft, very elastic black silicone tube for the penis, but also has a cord with silicone anal beads that can be inserted in her butt for the extra added "ding."

These items are available at a number of online sex toy shops.

eptember

how many things
can you do at once?

1 I go along with the generally agreed-upon principle that doing two or three things at a time when making love is better than just one. Yes, even when that one thing might be pretty great all by itself.

When a man is massaging the woman's clitoris with his tongue, for instance, he can be running three fingers below it with one hand, while fondling a breast with the other. If his tongue is active *below* her clitoris, he can even use his nose to stimulate her a little higher up.

As she is giving him oral sex, she not only uses her lips, but licks him with her tongue. Meanwhile, she can fondle or gently tug and twist his sack with one hand, while massaging his perineum—just behind his sack—with the other hand.

How do I love thee? Let me count the ways...

the put-on **rose**

2 We already considered the beautiful glass dildo with an embedded, frosted red rose. And the red rose that's really a teasing feather tickler. What else can they do with roses?

Make them into *panties!* And these are really cute, too. They look exactly like a rose, including the wrapping. But open them and they're panties. A great little gift for any romantic occasion. In red or white from *www.store1.yimg.com.*

---

russell crowe **sex**

I think of this as gladiator sex, because it looks like one combatant (the man) has bested the other (the woman), and is now taking his reward—on the field of battle. There are elements of sexism here, assault even, not to mention the possibility of groin strain, neck strain, and dizziness. What more could you want?

She's on her back, on the floor. (This won't work on a bed; you'll lose your balance.) He lifts her up by the hips and thighs and places her left leg across his chest, her foot resting on his left shoulder. Her right leg is bent at the knee, turned toward her breasts.

The victorious gladiator stands over her. His right leg is stretched to the back, while his left leg is placed between her legs. His foot is flat on the ground, close to her head. To help hold her lower torso in an upright position, his right hand supports her left butt cheek. His left hand is on his own left knee to support himself.

The woman may need pillows. And you may want to practice before carrying out the deed in the heat of passion. Finishing touch: gladiator outfits!

provocative fact #8
take tea and see

4 After drinking tea, Japanese researchers found, your arteries are more relaxed, and there is greater blood flow—both essential to good sex—for at least 2 hours.

---

the clitoris
as an iceberg

5 The clitoris is a pretty small organ to play such a crucial role in a woman's enjoyment of sex, isn't it? Even though it can swell up to nearly twice its normal size at the height of sex, it's still pretty diminutive. Some men have a hard time even *finding* it, let alone entertaining it. I never heard of a woman who had difficulty finding the head of a man's penis, which is the embryological twin of her clitoris.

Well, the clitoris, new research is showing, is like an iceberg: What you see is only about one-tenth of what's deeper down and hidden from view.

Doctors Jennifer and Laura Berman, in *For Women Only*, cite new work strongly suggesting that the clitoris we all know and love is intimately connected with tissues extending as much as 6 inches into a woman's pelvis, and is also "networked" with her G-spot and other areas of the vagina. The whole (perhaps we should say "holistic") clitoris, they claim, is longer than a man's penis. What's more, it becomes engorged and hardened during sex, just like a penis, even if less obviously.

No wonder more than half of all women report they rarely or never climax without direct clitoral stimulation. It's a lot more than a little button, just as its counterpart, the head of a man's penis, is a lot more than a little mushroom.

As the poet said, "No clitoris is an island."

---

groovin' in the groove

If you're the kind of person who believes that sex without penetration isn't sex, then this isn't sex. It's *better* than sex. At least if slow, spot-on teasing turns you on.

With the man in a state of reasonable firmness, the woman lies on top of him, her legs spread fairly wide. His small head is pointing toward his big head. Pressing against him, she very slowly slides up, then down, massaging the bottom of his penis with her vaginal lips. As they both rise to the occasion, she can include direct contact with her clitoris.

When her lips become sufficiently open, his penis will be "in the groove," as opposed to her vagina proper. Before she becomes wet, you may want some water- or silicone-based lubricant, possibly for both.

You can stay in the groove as long you like, but you'll probably choose to segue into groove number two or three.

meet me
after choir

The brain's "orgasm center" is located in its right prefrontal cortex, as we mentioned before. It turns out that both singing and dancing can pump voltage into the same general brain area.

I doubt that many people have sung or danced their way to orgasm—though some seem to be trying—but it's worth knowing these two cultural activities can serve as a kind of pre-warm-up. Perhaps this is why the two things grumpy old men hate most is singing and dancing. And another good reason for the two of you to go out dancing together, go to choir, or, like my wife, watch *Chicago* for the umpteenth time.

---

a new use
for old clothes

Not good suits or dresses, mind you. Those should be donated to Good Will. Besides, tearing off a guy's suit in bed is extremely difficult.

'Cause that's what you're going to do: Tear off, *rip off*, your lover's old T-shirt, ratty tank top, raggedy underwear, and beaten-up bra. Go at it together; first one to get the other naked wins. Giggling and screaming encouraged (don't try this just after you put the kids to bed).

To tell the truth, it helps if you cheat a little by snipping a bit here and there with scissors beforehand—collars and whatnot can be highly resistant to even the most passionate tugging!

the magic power
of your hands

9 A strange, sneaky kind of study was conducted some years ago in a library, of all places. As one group of people checked out their books, the librarians—having received their instructions—made subtle, fleeting hand contact with the clients as they handed them their cards or books. The other group of people went untouched.

Outside the library, the researchers conducted a "survey" about satisfaction with the library service. They found that way more people who had been touched rated the service as "excellent." They were the happy but unwitting recipients of secret "hand jobs."

When neuroscientists draw maps of the brain, showing the size of areas that are related to different body parts, the fingers and hands occupy a relatively huge amount of space, totally out of proportion with the size of these organs. So you can see why we are so exquisitely sensitive to being touched on our hands. If you want to flirt with someone, there is no better way than to "accidentally" brush your hand against theirs. If you happen to be married to that person, you shouldn't forget this lesson.

Holding hands is probably the most underrated of all loving gestures. Do it more often, every chance you get. It's even romantic if you're both wearing gloves. When combined with a nice walk together, the effect is multiplied; it's not just endearing, but proven to reduce stress and its harmful effects. Long hugs, in which your hands are holding or gently massaging your partner's, have a similar effect.

---

the well-dressed
penis

10 A standard accoutrement for today's stylish penis is a thin, stretchable sleeve covered with little bumps or doohickeys—even little soft spikes—to stimulate the woman's vaginal lips and wall. They're usually sold in sets of six or more, each with a different texture. A few have texture on *both* sides. Most can also be slipped over the fingers for use in manual pleasure-giving. Available from a great many sites offering sex aids.

provocative fact #9
who enjoys cunnilingus most?

11 In a survey of thousands of men and women, all over the age of 50, it was discovered that men enjoyed making oral love to their women more than the women enjoyed receiving it! Surprised? I sure as hell was! But there's a reason for this odd fact. When interviewed, the women said they would enjoy receiving oral sex a lot more if their partners a) went slower and b) were more gentle.

Moral for men: Don't be such an eager beaver if you want her beaver to be eager, too!

One more thing: The women also said they'd be a lot happier if their man shaved closer!

the
lipstick touch

12 Queried on their bedroom preference, many men say that lingerie is a great turn-on, but they also note that wearing sexy makeup can be an effective libido-raiser. Regardless of whatever else you're wearing or not wearing, try putting on a really dramatic, high-gloss, red lipstick. Start with his mouth and work your way down, all the way down. He will get very excited seeing your red lips working on him, especially with the lipstick stains on his penis.

---

believe it or not #6
the world's most expensive dildo

13 I imagine most people who own dildos take some pains to keep certain other people from finding them. But those who own the Huge Mr. Blue may actually put it in their will: It costs $900!

Made of handsome curved glass with embedded blue veins, this piece of modern sculpture is all of 16 inches long and has a serious-looking notched head on its shoulders. If you're on a budget, or 16 inches frightens you, there's a 10-incher available for only $750, from *www.domepuppy.com*.

---

pump up your sex life
with a blood pressure cuff

14 You may have noticed throughout this book that many things that are good for your health are good for your sex life, and things that are bad for your health have additional bad effects on your sex life. Here's another example that may surprise you: *High blood pressure can lower your sex drive.*

Tests have shown that men whose blood pressure is normal (120/80) have sex 25 percent more often than men with high readings. You may think that's because high blood pressure worsens the effects of high cholesterol, leading to artery disease. Probably so, but there's more to the story. High blood pressure actually reduces your testosterone! Low testosterone, in turn, can rob both men and women of sexual desire.

That's another reason to get a blood pressure cuff on your arm and check your reading. By lowering your pressure, you can literally pump up your sex life.

Consult with your physician, and be sure to discuss the sexual side effects of medications, because many of them, ironically, impair sexual performance. Discuss trying to first lower your pressure naturally, through weight loss, cutting back on salt, moderate exercise, and other means.

On the nutritional front, a major study identified the combination of low-fat dairy products and fruit as being especially helpful. And blueberries may be a very good choice to have with low-fat milk or yogurt: They're extremely high in antioxidants and are even recommended as a food that helps older men with erectile problems.

blind man **buff**

15

One or both partners blindfold themselves and then bumble around the bed or the whole bedroom (cleared of sharp-edged furniture). If just one partner is blindfolded while in the buff, the other can play hide-and-seek with the other, squirming away at the most teasing moments.

You can also pretend to get various body parts confused as a result of visual impairment, and try doing something different with her wrongly identified "mouth."

---

shock sex #5
give the full monty

16

Sometimes you need to let it all hang out. Usually, that may be in the final moments of your striptease or come-hither act. But doing the famous "Full Monty" when he or she is not exactly expecting it can create a special shock power.

She's reading a book and suddenly there's a bookmark of a kind she's never seen before pointing at the sentence she's on. Or he's into a newspaper when suddenly the sheets get pulled back and the Bermuda Triangle of Love is staring him in the face.

One minor problem is getting it out in one quick, smooth move. Her problem is over in a second with a break-away thong. Snap two little clips and the thong is headed for the floor. For him, there's a black leather thong with a yank-down front zipper. One yank and you're free! Both available from *www.flirtylingerie.com*.

---

undress
and de-stress

17

Feeling stressed is one of the most powerful anti-aphrodisiacs around. There are many ways to reduce stress, but here is the quickest way I've found.

Get undressed. Lie down. Take a slow, deep breath. Let it out slowly. For the next few minutes, continue this classic technique. You don't really have to count your breaths, but if you want to, six or seven per minute is best. Should you be thinking of anything in particular? Yes, your breathing, and nothing else. In... out... in... out. Not very profound thoughts, but it has a profound effect on your perceived stress. In as little as 2 minutes, you'll feel much more relaxed.

And it's not a bad idea for both of you to do this together. I don't advise coordinated breathing at this point; it takes your concentration away from relaxing your own bodies. Team breathing is best used during intermissions or transitions in lovemaking, or in the afterglow part of sex.

---

my darling **dildo**

18 A man and his partner can get good results if he begins by making many shallow thrusts into her rather than plunging right in to the deep end of the pool. The woman can reciprocate by using her man as a sex tool. She seizes hold of him at the base of his penis, and uses it to excite herself in the manner of her choosing, taking as long as she likes.

She may even want to shift her grip up higher on him, to stiffen his head and gain more control over it. She lets go of him when she's good and ready or when his batteries go dead.

the over-40
super-sex food

19

A friend of mine recently went to his doctor, who examined lab results and told him, "Looks like the Lipitor is really working; your cholesterol is great!"

Somewhat hesitantly, my friend admitted that he'd never filled the prescription; instead, he'd been using flaxseed.

Research shows that the higher a man's cholesterol, the more likely he is to have sexual problems, because his arteries are clogged. It's likely the same is true for women.

Flaxseed is relatively new to the health-food scene, and it deserves much wider use, for several reasons. For one thing, it's tremendously rich in the plant form of omega-3 oils, which are highly beneficial to the heart and circulation. Normally, oily fish like salmon or herring are recommended as a source of omega-3's, but just 2 tablespoons of flaxseed have 50 percent more omega-3's than a serving of salmon.

Those same 2 tablespoons also have 4 grams of fiber—as much as a whole cup of oatmeal!

What's more, flaxseed is fanatically high in antioxidants known as lignans, which have a very powerful health-promoting effect, including anti-cancer potency.

One magazine commented that while it's good for you, flaxseed "tastes like dirt." That is absolutely false; in fact, it tastes nutty, and when I add my 2 tablespoons to a bowl of high-fiber cereal—my current favorite being Optimum Zen—the taste is terrific. Maybe the brand I use is the secret: Try Bob's Red Mill Whole-Grain Flaxseed Meal and see if you agree. Not at your store? Visit *www.bobsredmill.com*.

Fantasy #9
seducing a stranger

20 Meeting some attractive person for the very first time and using all your powers of seduction to lure them into bed, might be immoral and even dangerous, but, let's face it, it can also be erotic in the extreme, leading to wild, uninhibited sex.

When the person you seduce is already your mate, the immorality and danger are gone, and all that remains is good, dirty fun. It's a fantasy you'll love, if you only try it!

There has to be a very specific fantasy scene for the seduction to be "real." Agree where it's going to occur: in the bar at the Half

Moon Bay Hotel; at the spa, with one person being the masseur or masseuse; at home, where the babysitter comes to the house for the first time; at the office of a female doctor, who gives an initial exam. Use your imaginations!

One person should take the lead, and the other be less forward. This is a *seduction*, remember. You've never seen one another before, so you have to go at it with appropriate decorum. Look each other over—slyly. Give each other compliments on little things like jewelry or shoes, or their taste in ordering wine. Ask all the questions you'd really ask if you were actually trying to ingratiate, relax, and flatter them. Slowly advance to light touches on the arm, brushing leg against leg, longer direct eye contact.

When the time is right you can either ask the seduced party to come to your hotel room, or perhaps to have sex right then and there, wherever that may be (her office, for instance). From beginning to end, the important thing is to never break the spell of the fantasy that you are making love for the first time.

If it "works out," you can make a date to meet again. Or try a whole different fantasy, with more devious flirting, or changing-of-the-mind teasing, surprise and shock, even ripping this and grabbing that.

sumo **sex**

21 In sumo wrestling, the combatants often stand directly in front of one another, and simply push for all they're worth. This next position is a little like sumo, because you're both standing, and pushing against each other, though the goal is different.

The man grasps and lifts one of his partner's legs as she stands before him. When her leg is positioned over his hip, he steps ahead with one leg and sets it down where the lifted leg was. He pulls her toward him until they are locked together. They take turns thrusting their loins, but take care not to push each other off balance. Very athletic, yet intimate at the same time!

sex
with your clothes on

22 Sex with your clothes on can be particularly erotic, especially if you're having a quickie. Some people find that pulling the panties to one side instead of removing them is also very provocative.

Here's a little trick to provide some foreplay when you're dressed. The man gets at her panties and begins giving her oral sex right through them. His mouth, tongue, nose all get into the act. So does his hot breath, which he blows through her panties. He circles around, too, kissing and nibbling her sweet bum.

She, of course, can do the same for him. It works best if he's wearing jockey shorts, but boxers will do in a pinch. She can put her whole mouth over his covered equipment and tease him by squeezing, licking, kissing, and giving him gales of warm, moist tropical breath. Don't let him drop his drawers until the discomfort—the outright *pain*—of his erection against his shorts becomes unbearable.

Fingernail **Finesse**

23 When I think of fingernails and sex, what comes to mind are long, red scratches on the back where your lover clawed you in the heat of feline passion. There is another place, though, where fingernails can come into play, only you'd better control the tigress in you, because it's the man's ball sack.

The scrotum of many men responds most gratefully to gentle nail scratching on the north-south axis. You can come down using the sharp tips, then stroke with the flat side as you go up. You have to gently pull his sack down with the other hand to create a proper playing ground.

Just above his pubic hair is another place that secretly craves the ministrations of a woman's nails. So does his whole groin area. So does… well, try it all over and see how he likes it. A whole-body fingernail massage is something special: even the fanciest spas don't offer it! Yet.

heat her up
in the oven

24 Back when I was a kid, we boys had to take shop class while the girls took home ec. While we hammered and sawed, they mixed and baked. One of their staple recipes was banana-nut bread, a pretty healthy cake compared to the other stuff they made. But banana-nut bread might be healthier than their teachers realized.

Inhaling the aroma of banana-nut, says smell expert Alan Hirsch, M.D., has been shown to increase both a woman's sexual arousal and her vaginal lubrication. It's the aroma, not the taste, so if either partner wants to bake a batch, it should be done while the woman is at home, and preferably within smell range of the oven.

While the aroma still fills your home, enjoy your cake with either coffee or tea. The caffeine in the coffee will perk you both up, while natural chemicals in the tea will make a man's arteries more flexible and able to dilate when blood begins to flow south.

Take some of the goodies upstairs with you.

sucking that
doesn't suck

25 A tongue caressing her vagina or clitoris is good, but many women get a bigger thrill from sucking, as opposed to licking. Alternate between one and the other. A woman can also try moments of sucking when giving a man oral sex.

sex
for bodybuilders

26 Having sex and sculpting your muscles at the very same time can be a special treat for anyone into well-rounded health—as well as those who are simply horny and vain. Here are two moves that build the upper body while the lower body gets its own workout. Either the woman or the man can do the first; the second is pretty much just for men—men who already have powerful arms.

The first move is nothing more complicated than a push-up, a familiar exercise that is still regarded as excellent for packing muscle on the triceps and pectorals. She (doing the push-ups) lies between his outspread legs, gets him inside her, and slowly presses herself up and down. Some adjustment of the position will be needed, and if desired, an extra element can be added if she rocks slightly this way or that at either the top or bottom of the push-up. Depending on your builds, both men and women may find it works better if the person on the bottom has a big pillow under their butt.

If the man (now it's him doing the push-ups) is *really* strong, he can add resistance by asking his partner to wrap her arms around his back. If he's really strong—a hell of a lot stronger than I am—he can even have her wrap her legs around his.

Having a push-up contest between lovers is not recommended; there will be the temptation to go up and down too fast to make it enjoyable. Also, unless your mattress is very firm, you may have to do this on the floor.

This next move is a good bit harder, and targets the triceps, the muscles under the biceps, which actually make up the bulk of the upper arm's musculature. The man sits on the floor, leans back, and supports himself with his hands. The most comfortable position is with fingers forward. His lover straddles him, supporting her weight both with bent knees and hands on the floor by his sides.

Now, here comes the hard part. As the woman lowers *some* of her weight on him, the man uses his bent arms as pistons to raise his butt—and his lover—off the floor. He slowly pumps his arms up and down, thrusting with the upward move. If more resistance is desired, the woman can lower more weight on him by leaning on him more, or widening the distance between her knees. The changing angles in this gambit provide different sensations, which can be very interesting.

The best part for some guys will be when someone at the gym asks how he got his triceps so ripped!

song of
the sarong

27 I love the sarong. It's sexy. Beautiful. Romantic. Comes in every fabric and design, from Indian to Hawaiian to African and Jamaican. It's the most versatile of all garments: Wear it on the beach or at the pool, coming out of the bath, entertaining friends, or just around the house to drive your man crazy. Cover just your hips, or your whole body. Wear it over sexy panties, a thong… or nothing.

The sarong doesn't scream its message: no, it's subtle, soft, natural… like *you*.

Years ago, Dorothy Lamour wore a sarong in no less than 15 movies, which established her as a preeminent sex goddess, and the sarong as the very icon of sultriness, *healthy* sultriness. Today, sarongs are enjoying renewed interest and many stores offer them in abundance. A good place to start is *www.allyouneedtowear.com*, where they have explanations of how to wear sarongs and how to tie them. Let him figure out how to *un*tie them!

sex
with flipper

28 Actually, it's like a dolphin and a *doughnut*. It's a dolphin because it's shaped like one, and fits over her vagina with a strap. It's a doughnut because there's a hole in the middle, where his penis fits. Flipper is a soft little guy who has a vibrator behind his head to stimulate her clitoris, and another one in his bottom to vibrate his testicles. Dolphins are very smart! (Diving Dolphin available from *www.intimategifts.com*.)

---

maybe he's not
such an animal

29 Many women have a notion that most men are somewhat animalistic, in the sense that they often initiate sex with little or no sweet talk or cuddling. Where's the *intimacy* that's so important?

Well, the intimacy *is* there, only it's on the other side of the sex equation.

"Men are about four times more likely than women to equate sexual activity with emotional closeness," writes Helen Fisher, Ph.D., in *Why We Love*. On the other hand, "Women report they feel more intimacy with a partner when they talk together just *before* making love."

Put a slightly different way, men are led to intimacy through sex; women to sex through intimacy.

This can have profound importance for your own love life. A woman may, for instance, get angry and really turned off when her man swoops down on her at home and cups her breasts. Or frustrated when he rolls on top of her in bed and pulls down her nightie without so much as a word. It's just his way of seeking intimacy.

I'm not saying men should not make a special effort to do more talking, cuddling, and neck kissing. They should. But a woman should understand that he's into intimacy just as much as she is. One survey, in fact, showed that the number-one thing men enjoyed most about sex was... *intimacy*.

You're both after the same thing, then, even if you're taking different paths.

rock-a-bye
your baby

30

This is a gentle, intimate "rock-a-bye-baby" technique you can enjoy in your bed, on a big sofa, even in a hammock. Lying side-by-side and fully engaged, you and your partner simply rock slowly back and forth. There's no pumping, no thrusting. Your bodies are continually touching from head-to-toe; that's the special appeal. Sweet and cuddly, and pretty much guaranteed to last a lot longer than more active trysting.

october

sex for
really serious
people

1 Are you the kind of super-intellectual person who continually reads books about the ultimate purpose of life, and then studies more books telling you how to achieve that ultimate purpose, with the result that you don't have enough time left to actually *do* that much? I know *I'm* not. But I think some people are, and if you are one of them, I imagine you might think that elevating *sex* to an art form, which we try to do in this book, perhaps seems beneath you. After all, how important in the grand scheme of things is a roll in the hay?

Well, listen to these words of a man called Aristotle, who was possibly even smarter than you: *"Happiness is the meaning and purpose of life, the whole aim and end of human existence."*

As we note elsewhere in this book, a direct and strong correlation has been found between sexual frequency and Aristotle's happiness: The more of one we experience, the more of the other we enjoy. Not that sex is *all* of the happiness pie, but it's a big, whipped cream–covered slice.

If Aristotle seems a bit ancient, consider the words of the current, 14th Dalai Lama: *"The purpose of our lives is to be happy."* He gets right to the point, doesn't he?

"Sex," some may think, okay; but what about naughty, even "weird" sex? Does that qualify as part of the Holy Secular Grail? According to another famous dispenser of wisdom, it does. In the words of Ts'ai Ken T'an, "Water which is too pure has no fish."

---

the joy
of jugs

2 Jesse Ventura, the sensational wrestler who went on to become governor of Minnesota, once said, "If I could be reincarnated as a fabric, I would like to come back as a 38-DD bra."

Needless to say, Ventura didn't say this in front of the state assembly, but in an interview in *Playboy*. And, although most men, in fact, are not that wild about really big breasts, it's undeniable that *some* are.

In the man-meets-big-boobs scenario, there are several points worth noting. One is that when a woman is lying on her back, her breasts tend to pancake out, even sliding over to rest on her ribs. This is not the most flattering configuration. It's better if the woman is on top, with her treasures bobbing over him. If she's supported on her hands, he will be able to fondle them; on her forearms, he can smooch them.

Having doggy-style sex in front of a big mirror can be doubly rewarding. He can not only envelop them with his hands but also watch himself doing it, which he'll love.

---

be politely
animalistic

3 There's a fine line between being animalistic and being an animal. Whenever possible, be more like the former. Though they may not openly admit it, most lovers don't want a bed partner who seems to have just stepped out of a Jane Austen novel. Of course, they don't want a brute, either.

Middle ground: When making love to her from behind, for instance, grab hold of her hair and gently tug it. Dr. Ava Cadell (whose Ph.D. is *not* in hair-pulling) favors this as an example of admirably "animalistic" sex.

ready, set...
ready, set...

4

In this position the woman look like she's getting ready to run a race, using the man's body as the starting block. He's on his butt, reclining backward. She's facing his feet, with her knees astride his thighs, and her butt over his loins. With him inside her, she uses her arms and hips to rhythmically move backward, as if getting "ready," then forward, as if getting "set." She has to pay attention and not commit a fault by slipping off his starting block.

provocative fact #10
why you're a fathead

5

Now that functional MRI can be used to map out brain activity, all sorts of things are being tested to determine their effect on our gray matter. In Great Britain, researchers have found that when people eat fat—as in ice cream or prime rib—their brain's pleasure centers are more excited than when they eat other, more healthful foods. Since the pleasure centers house the sexual centers, it seems like fat-free Fig Newtons are not good hors d'oeuvres to serve before sex.

They even went so far as to see if they could fake the brain into turning up the pleasure center by feeding it engineered feels-like-fat-but-it-ain't food. The brain called their bluff.

mutual
bondage kits

By its very nature, restraint always involves more than one helpful item. While you could quite easily provide many items from stuff around your house—scarves, undies, tape—you are better off buying a kit, if for no other reason than fiendishly tickling your lover with the same feather duster you use to dust your tabletops is not the most appealing thing in the world.

A basic but classy offering is the Prisoner of Love Restraint Kit. Classy because the four Velcro-closure arm and leg cuffs are lined with fur and satin, and the blindfold is also a sexy black satin. The restraints have straps to tie around your bedposts. (Available from *www.store1.yimg.com.*)

The Sexy Slave Kit is quite similar in concept, only everything is red instead of black, and no satin. But you do get a "pleasure feather," good for relentless removal of dust from body parts.

The Lovers Prison Kit is not very different except in one respect: The feathers are attached to a serious-looking rubber whip handle. You can give him 20 strokes of the cat-o'-nine-tails, but it'll feel more like a kitten. (Both available from *www.dear-lady.com.*)

---

the world's most
underrated sex food

7

It's not an aphrodisiac, because no one has yet shown that it puts you in the mood, but what it does do is put you in the pink as far as actually having sex goes.

The food is nothing more exotic than grapefruit. White or ruby red (my favorite).

What university-based research has discovered is that eating just one grapefruit a day reduces the artery-narrowing process by an amazing 46 percent. It's this artery business that impairs the potency of millions of men, and also harms many women's sex lives.

Now that your arteries are working better, consider this additional discovery: That same grapefruit, eaten on a daily basis, increases your energy level some 43 percent!

Not that other foods can't also improve your sex life, but this level of improvement in the resources you need for great sex is pretty hard to match.

Got grapefruit?

let me
rock you

There's something mysteriously comforting about a rocking chair. And something mysteriously pleasurable about rocking-chair sex. You can enjoy it with her facing either him or the cotton fields (if you're on the porch). The slow, rhythmic changes of pressure are delightful, and because you're both seated, there's a natural disposition to take it real slow.

Armless rocking chairs are the best way to go. They're not common, but we found a very nice one at *www.rocking-chairs.com*.

Called the Guitar Rocker because it's popular with guitarists (also nursing mothers!), it's made using Shaker joinery techniques and has a comfortable scoop seat. Gives the word "joinery" a whole new meaning!

---

the best way to
put her in the mood

This is going to surprise you. It surprised me, until I thought about it. Because it not only puts *her* in the mood, it works on *me*, too.

Can you guess the secret?

It's sex.

A great many women, says Rosemary Basson, M.D., *only* get "in the mood" after lovemaking commences. For them, the mood doesn't lead to sex; sex leads to the mood.

This observation has important implications. Consider: You're both lounging around, and one partner says to the other, "You in the mood?"

Reply: a shrug.

"Me neither."

End of discussion; end of opportunity.

Better to initiate some smooching, rubbing, groping. Even if both partners aren't initially "in the mood," they may find they are in a couple of minutes. And once they get between the sheets, the mood that wasn't there is suddenly making them voracious for sex.

Another way to look at this is that when someone says they're not "in the mood," it doesn't mean they wouldn't like to *get* in the mood. At the moment, they're kind of in neutral. In 10 minutes, they could be doing 75.

juice **her**

10

With a juicer, naturally. The Ribbed Juicer is a dildo, made of nubbed glass, and shaped just like an old-fashioned juicer, including the ribbed head. If that's not different enough to get her attention, there's a knob at the base, so the whole unit can be rotated to "juice" her! (Available from *www.doc-johnson-sex-toys.com*.)

let your lover
be your gps

11

Don't just *let* her, insist on it! Here's how:

The man (assuming he's in the "driver seat") begins his body tour in a certain spot, and after a time, asks her where she'd like him to go next.

"Wherever you like," she'll probably answer.

"I'm not going anywhere else until you tell me where," he replies. *Lovingly.*

At first she thinks it's funny, but pretty soon she'll get tired of him doing his thing at Twin Peaks and suggest he move on to the Lewis and Clark Trail, or wherever. Only he pulls the same stunt there after a while: "Where to now, my hot little GPS?"

The point: He forces her (sweetly!) to show him where she likes it, how long she likes him to visit each area, and where a good next stop might be. If the woman has been reluctant in the past to provide him with such invaluable guidance, now she has to get over it, or leave him stranded on the getting-sore-already Twin Peaks.

Tip to men: Don't begin with a foot rub; she may be glad to leave you there for a half-hour.

When the man is the GPS for the woman's tour, she must demand driving instructions from *him.*

TIP: **Don't start with oral sex; it'll be the shortest trip you ever took!**

fantasy #10
(i'm going to get in trouble for this)

12

NATIONAL AMERICAN INDIAN DAY

The second Monday of October is, according to every American calendar, Columbus Day, and we're getting close by now. No, I am not going to have Columbus Day sex! In fact, my calendar does not even have Columbus Day, as you can see. Instead, I choose to celebrate National American Indian Day.

This substitution has been urged by numerous Native American groups, and the state of South Dakota has taken the lead by changing the name of the holiday in their state. The justification for this is so obvious that I won't bother to explain it.

So, let's consider the fantasy of Native American sex, a prospect brightened by the observation of many early European settlers that the native inhabitants were exceptionally clean, well-groomed, physically attractive individuals. In other words, *hot*.

The really cute Indian Girl costume has a fringe dress, with lace-up sides, a feather headpiece, even a toy tomahawk she can threaten you with if you don't use that forked tongue of yours with the proper zeal.

A much more expensive outfit, but one that is really gorgeous, sexy, and will last a long time, is the Geronimo Fringe costume, made from suede, woven beads, and natural plumes. Find both outfits, with luck, at *www.trashy.com*.

go to the gym,
then to him

13

I mentioned before that after exercising, a woman's testosterone level is raised, boosting her sex drive. In case you think I said that just because I'm an exercise nut, here's some clinical, and I mean *clinical,* proof.

Sexual response researchers wired up women volunteers in such a way that changes in their vaginal swelling could be measured while they watched naughty movies. The first time, they screened the movies *then* asked the women to have an exercise session. The second time, they did the reverse: first exercise, then the movies.

Result: When the women watched the hot movies *after* exercising, their sexual response was two to three times greater than when they watched the films first!

Now, substitute sexy partner for sexy video, and the moral is clear: gym, then him.

Food that turns men into women

14 The higher a man's cholesterol level, the greater his chances of having erectile dysfunction. University researchers discovered this unsettling fact after examining the medical records of thousands of men.

Now, what causes high cholesterol levels? Besides genetics, it's eating lots of fatty foods. Or eating almost *anything* at Outback. The surprising thing is how quickly eating a fat-laden meal affects a man's love chemistry.

At the University of Utah, researchers gave men a rich milkshake, and discovered that in just a few hours, their testosterone was taking a nosedive, going down by a quarter or more!

This is a different phenomenon than being overweight— mentioned before—because *even a thin person* can be de-testosteroned (at least temporarily) by scarfing down the burger-bacon-cheese-bloomin' onion-huge steak-and-fries cuisine that is now so commonplace.

Consider cholesterol-lowering drugs if you must, but natural is better, and not just because it's cheaper. Some of these medications actually lower sexual prowess along with cholesterol!

never throw away
old scarves

15 They're good for many things in the bedroom, even on warm nights. Especially hot nights. Try wrapping one around the top of his scrotum, firmly but not *too* firmly. Slide it down so that his balls look like bulging breasts. Kiss and lick him the way you like your breasts treated.

You can also wrap the scarf around both his scrotum and penis when giving him oral sex. Again, firmly but not really tight. This will tend to keep him harder. There are sex aids that do the same thing, but a silk scarf is more romantic. An especially good idea if you want him to buy you a new one as a gift!

Frosting on
your cakes

16 While there's no shortage of purpose-made edible creams and body paints, one stands out as truly exceptional. Body Butter tastes and feels *exactly* like a delicious creamy cake icing! It's truly amazing. Frost whatever body cakes you like and dig in. Adds a whole new dimension to "oral" sex! Widely available in sex shops and sex aid Web sites.

---

shock sex #6
use hawaiian magic on her

17 If you're like me and some other men, you can literally shock your sweetheart with a sudden display of romantic charm and sensitivity. And there's nothing I personally find more romantic, even sensitive, than a Hawaiian lei.

Make a surprise appearance wearing little more than a lei around your own neck, and slip another one over her neck. "Feel like getting lei'd?" Corny, but effective. Especially if you're wearing a sarong!

You can find fresh leis and silk leis easily by putting "Hawaiian leis" into your browser. I think *www.royalhawaiianleis.com* is especially nice.

beef—
it's what's for sex

18

Well, maybe.

The protein in a steak will boost not only testosterone but also dopamine and norepinephrine, two natural chemicals in the brain that boost sensitivity during sex, says Elizabeth Ward, a registered dietitian and nutrition consultant. She also says, as quoted in *Men's Health* magazine, that beef *lowers* yet another chemical that tends to retard blood flow to the penis.

Now, a hefty, steakhouse-size slab of meat can have a metric ton of fat. And other studies show that feeding men big shots of fat can actually *reduce* testosterone. One university study showed that a few hours after slurping down a rich milkshake, men's testosterone levels had been pounded down by nearly one-quarter.

The solution seems to be that when enjoying your steak, a) choose a lean cut, like a tenderloin, strip steak, or eye round, and b) keep your portion size down to no more than about 4 ounces. That is only about half the size of most steaks, and even less if compared to a steak at contemporary steakhouses. Plus, most of those restaurant steaks come with big portions of French fries, not to mention onion rings and other infusions of fat. So c) is: Take a doggy bag home with you!

the boy scout
trick

19 When I was a Boy Scout, there was a test you had to pass in order to get promoted to Second Class Scout. It consisted of starting a fire by rubbing two sticks together. That's why I never got any higher than Tenderfoot. Later, however, I discovered you *can* start a fire by rubbing things together, albeit not sticks.

The woman can lie over her man as he makes a fist and places it above his penis. By slowly rubbing herself on it, she will become excited. (This can be done during actual intercourse as well).

In his excellent book *Great Sex*, Michael Castleman has these two suggestions for getting the first sparks to fly. The man places his arm between the woman's legs, holds on to her bottom with his hand, and positions his wrist or forearm so that it's against her vagina. She grinds against it.

Another move is for the man to place the heel of his palm over her mound and let her grind against it, while his fingers play on her vaginal lips, but don't purposefully open them. Both are good opening gambits. You may not see flames leaping out, but there should be some good honest smoldering.

what really makes a woman happy?

20 What brings the greatest sense of enjoyment to a woman? Having a really good marriage... a really good job... a perfectly clean house?

None of the above.

The correct answer is sex—sex and/or intimate relations.

This important fact is not from some rinky-dink survey, either, but from a study of 900 women conducted by researchers at the University of Michigan and recently published in *Science*, regarded as the world's most prestigious scientific research journal.

The authors suggest that while many may think that things like a secure job or a good income are major definers of happiness, it's what a woman actually *does* that brings her enjoyment. The least enjoyable thing, by the way, turned out to be commuting, with working just behind.

Give a woman her favorite things—sex and intimacy—when she gets home after enduring the worst: a day at work and the long drive home.

a gourmet guide
to edible lubricants

21 The folks at *www.ShopInPrivate.com* recently tasted and rated a few dozen edible lubricants and reported the results on their Web site. Some not only have flavor but also cause a sensation of heat if you blow on them.

As a fan of Diet Sprite, I was pleased to see that Motion-Lotion lemon-lime got a high rating; so did the same brand's High Passion (which also got a high heat rating). The overall winner among brands, however, was Wet, which offers a variety of flavors, including piña colada. The site offers a sampler package of a bunch of different flavors.

---

a few funny things
about viagra

22 One funny thing—and by funny I mean odd, not hilarious—about Viagra is that it isn't, as many suppose, a kind of aphrodisiac that fills a man with lust. It works, rather, by relaxing the smooth muscles in the penis, so that enough blood can flow in to create an erection. At least two similar drugs, Levitra and Cialis, work the same way. None have any effect on your brain, mood, or how fetching your lover appears. Without erotic stimulation, taking them is like putting premium fuel in a car that has no spark plugs.

Moral: Don't deny yourself the satisfaction such medications can bring because you feel there's something "unnatural" about them.

Another funny thing: Though it's easy to imagine that taking Viagra every time you have sex may leave you with a dependence on it, that doesn't seem to be true. In fact, it's been found that men who take Viagra on a daily basis over a period of months are often able to stop taking it (at least for a while) and still get good erections.

Theory: Your arteries have in some measure been rejuvenated by the fresh flow of blood through tissue that had been atrophying for want of nourishment.

A *really* funny thing about Viagra is that at least one research study has shown it to be notably effective in helping men who ejaculate too quickly to hold out longer! In fact, it worked better than an antidepressant frequently prescribed for this problem. The medical researcher said he had absolutely no idea why Viagra should work in this seemingly paradoxical way: "It just does."

Viagra is not approved for women as I write this; it's likely that some version of it might soon be, since the poor blood flow to the pelvic region that can leave men with potency problems can have almost equally harmful effect on women. Some women I know who have taken Viagra on their own initiative report that it boosted their sexual experience by 3 points on the Richter Scale. Whether this was physiological or psychological, I can't say.

In case you don't know it, you should *never* take these medications without a doctor's prescription. The major danger is that if you're taking nitrate heart medication, there could an extremely dangerous, even fatal, reaction.

Fantasy #11
the instant dungeon

23 Mutual bondage is probably most often enjoyed on a bed, with the recipient in a spread-eagle position. That can be accomplished by having him or her simply gripping the top bedposts and spreading their legs. If you're truly getting into it, though, you will want to use either silk scarves or soft Velcro wrist and ankle restraints that are attached to all four bedposts. The spread-eagle posture, by the way, provides the best access to most of the body's erotic zones and orifices.

Should you want something more advanced to act out your fantasies of restraint, one problem that pops up is the difficulty in tying someone against a wall, unless you feel like installing hardware into studs. That problem has now been licked with Door Jamb Cuffs. This is a set of four adjustable wrist and ankle restraints attached to straps that magically fit instantly on any door. No drilling or tell-tale iron cuffs mysteriously popping out of the woodwork! Practice interrogation techniques or do what you will on your new doorway to mutual bondage excitement. Not recommended for use on front door! (Available form *www.bettersex.com*.)

don't try this
in yoga class

24 Here is a position much honored in ancient India, home of yoga, the practice of which will help you remain comfortable during the act. If not, the position itself will give you a good gentle stretch, especially in the groin, thigh muscles, and low back.

The woman lies on her stomach with her knees flat against the bed. She reaches down and grasps her feet, wrapping her palms over the tops of each foot. She then pulls her feet up close to her butt, and at the same time angles them out to her sides, around her hips, as far as comfortably possible. Her partner then moves behind her, raises her thighs up, and slips his knees under them (or uses cushions).

When inside her, he slowly rocks back and forth, finding the angle and motion most pleasurable to both.

This is a very passionate position, which is described in a 15th-century Indian sex guide called the *Ananga Ranga*. And I am not going to tell you the name they gave it.

You insist on knowing, you say? Very well; it translates from the original as "Attack of the Tiger."

---

the
whole duck

25

"Kinky sex involves the use of duck feathers. Perverted sex involves the whole duck." —**Lewis Grizzard**

Do you feel a bit embarrassed at the thought of using some of the numerous sex toys and aids discussed here? Please do not deny yourself the fun and enjoyment these gadgets offer on that account; they are actually quite tame, middle America, middle-class pleasures.

If you want some idea of how relatively respectable they are, consider some of *these* sex-toy-oriented interest groups. (I'm not saying that what they enjoy is "perverted;" it's hard to describe any sexual act between consenting adults with that word. But they are, shall we say, more "technical)."

Electrosex: Sexually excited by receiving serious voltage from an impressive array of devices that look like they belong in Dr. Frankenstein's laboratory.

Pony Sex: Enthralled by everything about the little horsies; enjoy wearing bridles, real pony tails, and assorted pony tack. Group activities favored. Possibly neigh during sex.

Veggie Sex: Excited by produce for reasons that have little to do with nutrition. Get off by inserting all sorts of vegetables into every orifice (except the mouth): bananas, cucumbers, carrots, eggplant, and celery (not stalks, *bunches*).

Orgasmatronic Sex: Enjoy having sex with industrial equipment that pumps away like a big stamping machine. Used by both sexes in different ways.

S&M Sex: Aroused by administering and/or receiving pain. Usually accompanied by elaborate restraining techniques that range from being hog-tied to being suspended from the ceiling. Lots of leather and metal. Responsible practitioners keep things like bolt cutters, hacksaws, even block and tackle handy, in case of the need to release the recipient in an emergency.

And the moral? Using the things we discuss in this book is only 21st century Ozzie and Harriet.

girding his
lascivious loins

26

Sexy things for *him* to wear are a lot harder to find than those for her. There are a few frolicsome undies, though, that may ring your bells—and his, too.

If you've ever wondered what a Scotsman looks like underneath his kilt, you can find out extra-fast with this smart-looking plaid kilt that covers nothing but his bagpipe. The T-Bar Kilt Thong, from *www.lingeriegifts.com*.

If he's a real stud, or thinks he is (all men *do*), you can acknowledge his prowess with a studded leather thong. *Very* manly!

Want something more on the playful side? Consider the pouch brief featuring the fake fur head of a dog—or elephant (well-hung, trunk-wise). All can be found on *www.store1.yimg.com*.

sweeten up a sourpuss
technique #2 the happy diary

27 Of all the psychology tips I've seen over the years, this is one of the best. Read it even if one of you isn't a sourpuss; it could still help enrich your life.

Researchers asked a number of people to keep diaries. One group was asked to record things that ticked them off that day. Another group was told to simply record what had happened that day. The third group was asked to record up to five different things that they felt thankful for that day.

After just 2 weeks, the thankful-for group was much happier than before. Not only more so than the ordinary diary-keepers, but happy enough that their spouses noticed a definite change in their attitude. Michael McCullough, Ph.D., one of the researchers, sees gratitude as a kind of tonic for both body and mind—making you not only happier, but more energetic. That's a good combination for a bed partner.

I'd suggest giving your partner a handsome diary and telling him (or her) the idea. Just to make it look less like a "therapy," it's best if you let your partner know you're *also* scribbling away each day. After a few weeks, compare notes over a glass of wine. You could have a wonderfully intimate—and revealing—experience.

> **BONUS:** A Johns Hopkins study has shown that people with a positive attitude are only half as likely to have a heart attack as negative types!

double
her pleasure

28 I doubt that even the most flexible yogi could have penile intercourse with a woman while giving her clitoris oral sex at the same time. To correct this notable failure in human anatomy, clever sex toy designers have come up with a chin harness that wraps around the head and accommodates a plug-in dildo of your choice (up to 3 inches in diameter). While the man's chin inserts and controls the motion of the dildo, his mouth is free to make love to her clitoris.

Okay, it's a little scary-looking (that's *good*), but it does a unique job. The best thing about one model, called The Accommodator, is one customer's review, which states, "I LOVED this contraption. My wife said it was like having sex with me and my brother only we didn't have to have him over, get him loaded up, and use him like the animal he is." (Available from *www.lingerietoys.com*).

---

the bondage duckie

29 This rubber ducky has two features not found in the one you played with as a kid—at least, I hope not. First, he's wearing a little bondage outfit, complete with spiked collar. Second, he's got a vibrator on board. And of course, he's waterproof and floats, so he won't drown when he goes down on you. (Available from *www.goodvibes.com*.)

even the best man
can't do this

30 With their vibrations, projections, and controls, sex toys meant for a woman's pleasure can outperform even the best stud—at least, technically. The greatest satisfaction comes from having sex toys and *him* working on you at the same time. Besides doing other things, he can participate by operating control mechanisms in such a way as to tease and surprise you. Here are a few examples of some dildos and vibrators that seem especially ingenious, often amusingly so, with magical powers that no man alone can provide.

A good example of a sex toy that is basically pretty simple but still notably different is the *inflatable* dildo. The one under my spotlight right now is black (most sex toys are pinkish), in a realistic penis shape, with a slight curve, and attached to a bulb pump. By squeezing the pump, you can fill the thick, durable rubber with more and more air, until its diameter is a full 3 inches. Then deflate. Inflate. (Available from *www.search.stockroom.com*).

Here's a toy that not only vibrates, but can be bent in any direction to convey its energy to whatever area of your body craves attention. Shaped like a realistic penis—some 8 inches long—and with a natural skin feel, the Robo Cock has no less than 10 speeds and five functions (including "Roller Coaster"). Either of you can work the controls. (Available from *www.extremerestraints.com*).

Imagine a penis toy that not only vibrates but also *heats up* and *lights up* on command. Called Shane's World Rechargeable Infrared Playpal, this is a real hoot—and holler. Waterproof, too (the one thing it has in common with a man!). (Available from *www. luckysextoys.com*).

Fantasy #12
sex with a witch

31

HALLOWEEN

Come Halloween, every man gets a strong urge to do two things: Eat at least a dozen Krackle miniatures and insert his penis into a witch. Especially a good-looking witch, with nice straight teeth.

If one doesn't fly through your window, you can turn your sweetheart into a saucy substitute by buying her a Sexy Witch costume. And it really *is* sexy: The all-black dress has a lace-up front that can be adjusted to cast a spell over you, turning you into a drooling dog. Comes with a high pointed hat and black fishnet hose. *Wicked!* (From *www.store1.yimg.com.*)

november

earn $50,000
tonight

What is your love worth to you, in dollars and cents? That would seem to be an absurd question, but nothing is too absurd for university scientists. Now, economists from England have found that you *can* answer such a question. Pioneering a field they bluntly call Happiness Economics, they cranked through tons of survey data (from Americans, not Brits). By comparing how happy these people said they were to other factors—like their sex lives and incomes—the economists reached several conclusions.

For one thing, having sex at least once a week (as opposed to infrequently) is worth $50,000 in money. In other words, it has the same power to increase happiness as being left 50 thousand bucks in uncle Otto's will.

A good marriage? That's worth $100,000.

And, oh, one more thing they discovered: The more sex someone has, the happier they are, on average.

Josh Billings, a sort of folksy proverb monger, once said, "Don't mistake pleasure for happiness. They are a different breed of dogs." That's probably true for pleasures like cigar smoking and gambling, but sex is proof that pleasure and happiness *are* connected—at the waist.

the body smell men love

2

It's the smell of eggs. Not poached eggs, not scrambled eggs: *your* eggs.

Scientists rounded up a bunch of guys in a laboratory and handed each one two women's T-shirts. Worn-all-day unwashed tees. Give 'em a good sniff, said the researchers, then tell us which tee belonged to the more attractive woman.

Suckered as usual in such experiments, the men did not know that the two shirts they were holding their noses to actually belonged to the same woman. The difference between the two shirts was this: One had been worn while the owner had been ovulating, the other when she wasn't.

Fully 75 percent of the guys chose the ovulated-in shirt as belonging to the more attractive woman. To put it in veterinary terms, it seems as though a fair number of men were subconsciously able to detect the smell of a woman "in heat."

Unless you're on the "rhythm" method, you might want to test out this theory by making it a point to snuggle up close and long with your man when you're ovulating, and not wash too much. Is he not interested? Remove various articles of clothing that have been in close contact with your skin, and hold them under his nose. Eventually, you'll wind up naked, so it might not matter if he's an "ovulation hound" or not.

---

the
switcheroo

3 Changing positions during sex is to be praised, but it's not done often enough. Here's a very easy way to switch gears, your only props being a low bed and a pillow.

She lies crosswise on the bed, face up, her legs over the side, feet planted on the floor. He kneels on the pillow on the floor, draws close to her, and enters her. This is really a variation on the "mish posish," but the angle is so different—more aimed at the G-spot—that it's a new experience.

Now the quick switcheroo. She simply rolls over, and presents her sweet ass to the man (still kneeling on his pillow), who enters her from behind—perhaps even changing ports of call.

no-brainer #3
be a loser to win more sex

Common sense tells us that when you trounce someone in a game, whether it's Monopoly or bocce ball, it's not going to help put your playmate in a romantic mood. Yet, many of us often can't resist the impulse to win. I'm sure you've met people who feel compelled to win at *everything*. But they could be losing something more important than a miniature golf game.

Researchers from the University of Plymouth, in England, actually studied this win-lose dynamic in a group of women and made two notable discoveries. One, their heart rate, upon winning, went up an average of 10 points, a big jump. More significantly, they told interviewers that winning made them *sexually aroused*.

So, are you man enough to lose?

my favorite
romantic touch

5 Men like romantic touches with three characteristics: 1) easy, 2) cheap, and 3) leading to sex. So you MUST buy this for Valentine's Day, her birthday, or your anniversary. The Bed of Roses is a collection of over 100 scented silk rose petals. Scatter them around a bath you've drawn for her, or on the bed of love. You'll still have enough left to lay down a rose-strewn path for her to follow. It comes with four candles; even a special invitation card. (Available from *www.bettersex.com*.)

last-second sex
tricks: **volume #2**

6 John Gray, Ph.D., the Mars-Venus guy, suggests that, just a second or two from when a man is ready to blow, his partner use a couple of fingers to firmly massage his perineum, the small area just below his scrotum and close to his prostate. I am of the opinion that the average guy will have a Mount St. Helens orgasm when his partner does this. The man could also try this on his woman and see is she also goes volcanic.

Another way to get to his prostate: Just a few seconds from blast-off, insert your longest finger (pre-coated with lubricant) into his bum hole. The pad of your fingertip is toward his abdomen. Slide up about 3 inches, hook your finger, and make "Come here" gestures as he writhes in ecstasy. This is one of the most intense sexual pleasures a man will ever experience.

testosterone for women? hmm...

By now, you know that testosterone (which used to be erroneously called "the male hormone") is crucial to the sex drive of women as well as men. Men who test low on testosterone are currently being prescribed patches that release the hormone into their bloodstreams. But what about women?

As I write, the U.S. Food and Drug Administration has just denied approval for a testosterone patch for women called Intrinsa. They said the maker had failed to produce sufficient evidence that the drug was safe and effective.

One medical commentator said that despite the developer's claims, their own tests showed that women (with low testosterone) who used the patch increased their frequency of sex from three times a month to five times a month, while women who used a placebo patch (with no active ingredients except the power of suggestion) went from three times to four times a month. So the net benefit was just one more sexual episode a month.

Perhaps by the time you read this, the requisite evidence will have been produced, and the drug might be available. Check with your physician.

---

shock sex #7

"i'll make you a deal"

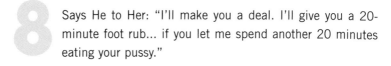

Says He to Her: "I'll make you a deal. I'll give you a 20-minute foot rub… if you let me spend another 20 minutes eating your pussy."

a six-star
submarine vibrator

9 Good Vibrations is one of the leading and most reputable sources of sex toys. This particular vibrator was actually designed by their own staff, to incorporate many of the requests received from customers. The G-Twist Vibe has a G-spot curve, a "clit ridge," a very erotic textured shaft, variable speed, and a "smooth, velvety body." And, oh yes, it's waterproof; perfect for when you want some extra steam coming out of your bath water! Comes in a really nice-looking Baby Blue and other colors, from *www.goodvibes.com*.

Fantasy #13
be all you can be

10 People have a million different fantasies, and we've only suggested a few so far. But there's almost no end to the possibilities for living out your fantasies with appropriate costumes from a Web site, at least if you're a woman.

You could, for instance, be a pirate's wench... Little Bo-Peep... a biker babe... Tinker Belle... a naughty nurse... a hillbilly... a police-woman or naughty prison inmate... Catwoman or Little Red Riding Hood. Two of the most unusual have to be a ladybug outfit... and a Drug Enforcement Agency get-up. Sex with a DEA agent? Yeah, I think about that *every day!* A very large selection of costumes can be seen at *www.trashy.com*.

If you're interested in the "bitch" look, visit a site like *www. erosboutique.org*, which has a wide selection of vinyl and leather costumes, many *extremely* erotic. Let me put it this way: You *won't* look like Little Bo-Peep!

in praise of
swallowing

11

This is very strange. But every man and woman, especially those who may have a baby in their future, should know about it. I would not, however, go so far as to recommend putting it on the refrigerator door as a reminder.

Women who perform oral sex on their mates and swallow his

semen—at least some of it—are notably less likely to suffer from a pregnancy complication called preeclampsia, in which blood pressure takes a dangerously high spike. It's theorized that the small amounts of sperm the woman ingests condition her immune system to accept the "invasion" of his genetic material without overreacting in pregnancy with life-threatening results.

Plus, it's been more recently found that sperm contains a certain molecule that actually boosts the effectiveness of a woman's natural killer cells, those invaluable defenders that do things like attack cancer in its very earliest stages.

All of which leads to the question of how sperm tastes. Generally, it has a somewhat bitter taste, though not *really* bitter. Some say that coffee and broccoli consumed the same day make the taste worse; apples are reputed to sweeten the taste. (Is *that* why they say, "An apple a day...?")

upside-down **sex**

12 Sometimes this happens spontaneously, especially if you like to wrestle around on the bed. Or you can purposefully put it on the menu.

With the woman on her back, the man lifts up her hips high

enough so that only her head, neck, and shoulders are on the bed. The rest of her body is supported against his chest. Depending on height and fitness, the man can either be kneeling or standing. He then makes love to her orally. Her blood will be confused because while it wants to flow to her lowered head, it also wants to go down (*up*, I mean!) to her vagina, where the action is.

Sex therapist and author Lou Paget is another aficionado of upside-down sex, and suggests that the woman should wrap her legs around the man's neck, locking her feet behind him.

This is a fitting position for the man who has lost a BWF (Bedroom Wrestling Federation) match with his lover. Or maybe he's won!

words as sex toys:
multiplying the effect

13

Some couples, while providing color commentary on their sexual union, use sweet, endearing, entirely positive words: "You're driving me wild... You're delicious... I'm in heaven!"

Others find that talking dirty is a strange and powerful excitant: "Your (fill in) is (or are) fantastic... Put that big (fill in) inside me *now*... I love to eat your (fill in)... (Fill in) me!!"

You may use one lingo one night and the other the next night. Best of all is to intermingle both during the same lovemaking session.

Whichever approach you take, you can greatly magnify the effect by holding your face close to your lover's and staring her or him right in the eye. Usually, when people talk during sex, they have their eyes closed. By keeping them wide open and looking directly into your partner's soul, it's a whole different experience. Most will find this very intense, though some, I suppose, will find it too intense, a kind of invasion of their sexual soul space. They can probably get over it in time, and may learn to treasure this new, higher level of intimacy.

the world's
most pleasurable
resistance training

14

We mentioned before under "The Ultimate Sexercise" that doing Kegels can strengthen the pelvic floor muscles and increase sexual pleasure. There are several devices you can use to provide resistance and measure the strength of your squeezes. Here is a slightly different approach to the same idea.

Suggested by therapist Barbara Keesling, Ph.D., the exercise is quite simple. With a dildo deep inside you, tighten your muscles as you would to do Kegels (basically, the same thing as stopping the flow of urine). Now, gently tug on the dildo, but resist with your muscles. Dr. Keesling advises that doing this exercise can make you "adept at gripping your lover's penis," which can feel fantastic for both of you.

sex over the internet

15 Your lover is in Portland, Maine; you're in Portland, Oregon. You email and IM each other every day. Now, you can take your long-distance love to the next step: Internet intercourse.

What makes this possible is something called the Televibe-Phone/Internet Controlled Sex Kit. A 7-inch-long, curved soft jelly vibrator unit is at the "receiving" end. Once connection is established by Internet (a touch-tone phone works, too), the person on the other end assumes control of the vibrator, and can send nine different instructions: pulse, super pulse, throb, buzz, and so on. Definitely not invented by Bill Gates! (Available from *www.extremerestraints.com*.)

melt her
with this candle

16 Green apple. That's one of best scents for melting away a woman's feeling of stress, according to Alan Hirsch, M.D., probably the world's leading expert on the effects of fragrance. If you can't find a tree with green apples, there are always candles and other fragrance-generating whatnots available. Buy a few different kinds and experiment over a few nights. If nothing else, it's a conversation-starter. ("Do you think 40 candles is too many?")

---

dear **sir:**

17 Please take a moment of your time to answer the following question: If you could choose just one position in which to *enjoy sex, from now until the* *end of time*, what would that position be?

When the researchers who asked this question tallied the results, they found that the number-one choice was "woman on top."

Surprised?

Maybe it's because men get a large charge out of pleasing their sex partner, and the woman-on-top position is surely one of the best routes to this reward. Famous sex researchers Masters and Johnson declared that only this position, and side-by-side sex, "allow direct or primary stimulation of the clitoris to be achieved with ease."

But it gets better, as most women know. Because it allows her to shift positions—moving forward and back, or from side to side—she has far more control than when she's under his body.

But she-on-top also has benefits for the man. For one thing—or two, actually—there are her breasts, just where he wants them. And breasts that are more or less pouring themselves into his mouth may be more exciting to him than ones that are just lying there, flattened against her chest.

Many men also say the stimulation of their penis when she's on top is a little less intense than when he's on top, the upside of which is they can last longer.

unsolved mysteries of
the sexual universe
part #2

male performance
anxiety

18

Everyone's heard of male performance anxiety: expected to be a stud muffin, he turns into more of a muffin because the "pressure is on." But some studies suggest that performance anxiety may be a figment of the imagination, perhaps covering up for other problems.

David Barlow, M.D., a pioneer in measuring sexual arousal through monitoring blood flow into the penis, showed two groups of men erotic movies. One group was given this warning: If they did not achieve a degree of arousal at least equal to the group average, they would get an electric shock. He was lying, of course, but they didn't know it; they expected to get a small version of the electric chair if they didn't get righteously hard. The pressure was on!

The second group of guys was shown the same porn flicks and not told anything except that their arousal would be monitored as a matter of scientific interest.

Any reasonable person would predict that the "pressured" group would not get as turgid as the second, but guess what? They got bigger erections! This suggests that a bit of a challenge may actually inspire men to greater achievement.

And are you ready for *this?* Researchers who investigated the rare cases where gangs of women held men at knifepoint and demanded sex, found that the men not only got it up, but did so *repeatedly!*

Now, I'm not suggesting that women should take a Henckels steak knife into the bedroom with them. But there are other ways of issuing a challenge that might bring out the most in your man. You could, for instance, tell him point-blank: "I want you to f... my brains out! That's an order!"

---

provocative fact #13
atkins, shmatkins!

A high-protein diet tends to lower testosterone levels. Reducing calorie consumption by more than 15 percent (around 300 to 400 calories per day) also lowers testosterone.

Moral: For sex sake, trim down with exercise, and eat salads dressed with "mono" oils—olive, canola, or peanut. Both approaches *raise* testosterone.

"Feeling naughty"
lingerie

20 Now, we're beyond the "playful" look... beyond the "sexy" look... at the door of the downright naughty look... the look that says... nothing in English: It just purrs, and growls throatily.

Besides some of the fantastically sexy bras we've mentioned (like the shelf-bra), there are any number of lingerie choices that can make any boy boisterous and any girl a pirate's wench.

Fishnet pantyhose and bodystockings are especially hot because they theoretically cover a lot of the body, but you can see right through them. Teasing works every time!

Thigh-highs are long stockings that stay put without garters: a different, almost refreshing look. And please consider *suspender pantyhose*, another novel look, in which pantyhose are cut to make it look like you're wearing separate stockings and garter belt. These ultra-hot numbers can be made even more provocative when they're worn without panties.

The *G-string* and the *thong* are both minimalist in the extreme, with the latter having just a few more molecules of fabric than the former. One style of G-string has a strand of pearls instead of a fabric front, attached to a lace waistband.

Crotchless panties don't have to be as obvious as they sound. While some models have visible open space, more modern models look like any other panty, but the front can be easily parted by eager hands or other body members.

---

fantasy #14
kidnapped!

21

A friend of mine has played this game with her husband for more than 30 years. A time or two every year, one "kidnaps" the other. Doesn't matter how much work they have to do, the "victim" must go along with the kidnapper without question or complaint. They drive off to an undisclosed location, with the victim trying in vain to figure out where they're headed. The destination is usually some really out-of-the way romantic bed & breakfast or country inn.

The kidnapper has everything prepared to pamper, soothe, amuse, and feed the victim, including a menu of sexual delights.

Beats staying home and watching *Without a Trace*!

turn your tongue
into a sex toy

22 Most vibrators are designed to directly pleasure some sensitive part of the body. There are a few, though, that do it indirectly, by turning your tongue into a sex toy. The Ultimate Oral Pleaser is a small vibrator encased in what's called Cyberskin. Attached to straps that loop around the ears, the devilish gizmo can be worn over or under the tongue to give it new powers of stimulation. Or, you can simply hold it between your lips and give a tactical massage.

The Tongue Joy is a more sophisticated and more aggressive tongue-booster that can be strapped around the tongue or other parts with the three different straps. It comes with silicone sleeves that do double-duty as stimulators and protectors of your pearly whites. (Both available from *www.bettersex.com*.)

the world's
sexiest outfit

23

Wear it on a romantic vacation... his birthday... Valentine's Day... your first or your 31st anniversary. Whenever, it's super-hot, and best of all, super-simple.

All it is: a long, extra-full, extra-large, high-quality red boa that you wrap around your otherwise naked body any which way you like. It's both fun and dazzling. You'll want to practice different moves in front of the mirror to come up with the most teasing, provocative ideas you can. Accessorize with a pair of stiletto heels to complete the totally devastating look. Fantastic choice for a long, torrid strip-tease! (Available from *www.lollipoplingerie.com.*)

head trip #2
"tell me a fairy tale"

24 Communicating directly about sexual fantasies is not the easiest thing in the world for many couples. Here is a way of sharing fantasies that makes it easier, at least if you're good at stream-of-consciousness talking.

Take a familiar fairy tale—*Little Red Riding Hood*, for instance—and take turns giving your own versions. The only rule is that your fairy tale has to be romantic, sexual, or both.

So Little Red Riding Hood went to Grandma's house to bring her some goodies. When she got there, the Big Bad Wolf was in bed, pretending to be grandma.

"What do you have in your basket for me, dear?" the wolf asked.

"Two chocolate bars, a bottle of Australian cabernet, and a pair of handcuffs," Red replied.

"Handcuffs?" said the wolf. "Whatever for?"

"Just watch me," said Red, as she slowly unbuttoned her blouse.

There could also be a more romantic version, where Little Red Riding Hood gradually develops a relationship with the wolf, who turns into a handsome prince after he gives Red a rousing round of oral sex.

Snow White and the Seven Dwarfs, Cinderella, Sleeping Beauty, Hansel and Gretel, and many other tales can all be used as screens on which to project your fantasies. If you think that all of this is outrageous, bordering on blasphemy (not to mention bestiality, pedophilia, etc.), so much the better!

thanksgiving **sex**

25 Thanksgiving is here, and many families are already getting together the ingredients for stuffing, cranberry sauce, pumpkin pie... and sex. Well, *some* are. Actually, that may very well include *you*—even if you don't know it!

An M.D. by the name of Alan Hirsch, who researches such things, has reported that a combination of the fragrances of pumpkin pie and lavender increased men's penile blood flow by an average 40 percent. Translation: hornier, harder.

If you're baking a pumpkin pie, you're halfway there. Get some lavender fragrance from an aromatherapy shop, and the spell should be complete. The good doctor also reports that cinnamon buns and doughnuts do a good job, too. So if you're too stuffed to think about love after Thanksgiving, you could bake *them* the weekend after, when the turkey should be nearly digested.

what i learned
from bambi

The first movie I remember seeing as a child is *Bambi*. I was *enthralled*. Thirty years later, however, I discovered that the Disney people left out an important part of the story: the part where Bambi performs cunnilingus on Fawn.

Let me explain.

Some years ago, when I had a house on a wooded hilltop, I awoke one rainy, sleety fall morning to see two deer not 20 feet from the side window. The doe was eating tips of shrubbery. The buck was eating *her*. And he was doing it with great gusto. As his long tongue did its warm-up work, her white tail was scooting back and forth a mile a minute.

I was dumbfounded. I mean, deer don't normally forage right next to an occupied house, let alone perform oral sex in front of a picture window, where there's a guy fumbling with a movie camera. But there they were.

Now, I didn't use a stopwatch, but I estimate that the buck spent between 5 and 7 minutes attending to her vagina. Only then did he mount her. The actual intercourse, as I recall, lasted barely a single minute.

I had to ask myself: Was there a lesson here? Two came to mind.

One was that the notion one used to hear years ago about oral sex being somehow "unnatural" was obviously wrong. If Bambi is doing it to Fawn, how much more natural can you get?

More important, perhaps, was the math. The ratio of foreplay to intercourse, that is. Which worked out to about 6:1, in favor of foreplay. In human terms, that would translate to about 3 minutes of intercourse (that's about the average time, sex researchers say) preceded by nearly 20 minutes of foreplay. Does that sound about right? John Gray, Ph.D., suggests 20 to 30 minutes, so I think we're close.

Is it totally wrong to draw lessons about human sexuality from Bambi? Probably, even though I agree with the lessons anyway. And besides, I *loved* that movie!

---

emeril lagasse
sex

27

Emeril, the entertaining chef, always likes to "kick it up a notch." In the late throes of passion, you may want to kick it up a notch, too, and maybe you should. As Dr. Alex Comfort notes, "Stimulus toleration increases with sexual excitement until even hard blows can become excitants (though not for everyone)." So, you may not have to restrain yourself from the wild thrusting, sucking, playful slapping, or whatever you're doing when the love lamp is on full flame.

But—I'm sure you've already noticed this—the doctor adds that this lessened sense of pain "disappears almost instantly with orgasm," so you have to back off immediately, and be extra-gentle, because many people become very tender within seconds of climaxing.

<hr />

wine
for the ears

28 Romantic music—there's tons of it. But *erotic* music is something else. While romantic music's mission is to make you soft and dreamy, erotic music is the next stage: what might be called perisexual music, meant to be consumed just before, during, or after sex.

The big difference is something very simple: lyrics. You almost automatically begin mentally singing along with the words to romantic music. Maybe you even think about the lyrics, how true they are, and all that stuff. All of which interferes mightily with what you really need: Something to help you focus on nothing other than your lover and your lover's hot body.

Searching through my collection of CDs—The Queen's Royal Pipers, Fatboy Slim, Gospel All-Stars—I discovered I definitely had nothing that could be construed as workable erotic music. So we ordered something that seemed like it couldn't miss: *Erotic Nights— Music for Making Love*, composed by John Gonzalez. We turned it on... and waited.

First reaction: This is the background music they play in movies during torrid romance scenes, and nearly all the time in soft-core adult movies. Lots of sultry sax.

Second reaction: Every track is more or less the same as the one before. There's no sense of building passion, like in Ravel's *Bolero* (which doesn't work, unfortunately, because you start laughing if you saw the movie *"10"*). There's no real melodic line, either, just meanderings. And that sax player, can't he go out for a weed break?

Third reaction: Oh my God, it's starting to kick in! But *why?* Main theory: I'm having a Pavlov's dog conditioned reflex—after years of listening to similar movie soundtracks that obviously mean pretty-soon-they're-gonna-do-it, my brain is starting to salivate. Subtheory: The very lack of musical line, and the repetitiousness of this CD, empties the mind of distracting thoughts, and fills it with... *sax* music. **Conclusion:** It *works*.

While we bought this CD from *www.bettersex.com*, Amazon has a collection of erotic music, with lots of samples. If it's still there, you may want to check out *Rhythm/Pleasure* by Rip Rowan.

a buzz for a
busy woman

29 While she's busy working, reading, or doing almost anything short of going for a run, she can give herself a buzz with any one of a number of hands-free vibrators worn under her clothing.

The She Shell is a pretty intimate little guy, designed to stimulate both vagina and clitoris, while concealed under clothing. It comes with a detachable, multi-speed control unit. (Available from *www.luckysextoys.com.*)

Another choice, with a somewhat less romantic name than the She Shell, is Vibrating Crotchless Panties, consisting of crushed velvet panties and a small vibrator. (Available from *www.store1.yimg.com.*)

erotic movies,
clean and dirty

30 One of the most common themes in many sex guides is that there exists a special kind of erotic film, made by and for women, and that these present sex "from the woman's perspective." This perspective includes a plot, relationships, and a slowed-down tempo of sexuality. They not only have a special appeal for women, but are also great for watching by couples. They are what might be called clean dirty movies. The one director mentioned over and over again as a producer of such movies is Candida Royalle, an ex-porn star turned moviemaker. Naturally, my wife and I ordered one, *Stud Hunters*, and watched it with high hopes.

I will not go into the 13 different reasons we found this to be the stupidest, most tedious, boring, inane, talent-free, and bizarrely *un*sexy movie we'd ever seen in our lives. As for the "woman's perspective," the final sex scene shows a woman going at it with four guys at once, although in remarks added to the film, the director remarks that "she's in charge," not the men.

But the same could be said of virtually every sex scene in *any* pornographic movie made in the last 20 years or so: Compulsion, or forced, sex simply does not exist, even in the raunchiest porn flick. The woman not only consents, she's usually the one who initiates the action.

We then rented what's called a "couples movie," which, although not as sensitive or female-oriented as Candida's films are supposed to be, is still the kind of movie a couple could watch together, even if it were their first time at it. We chose a film called *First Class*, and found it much better, and sexier, than the Candida flick.

Then, there are traditional XXX-rated movies that don't pretend to be anything other than sexually exciting. If the couples approach doesn't work for you, you should try them. Though some complain that what they depict is unrealistic, the same could be said of the majority of mass-market films, with their presentations of crime, violence, amazing escapes, and other things we're unlikely to encounter in real life—especially aliens. Who wants to watch a movie—sexual or not—that looks exactly like what you did last night?

One way to obtain X-rated films is to rent them from a place such as *www.BushDVD.com*, where for a monthly fee, they send you your choices from a library of over 13,000 titles. They say you can drop out any time if you're not happy.

December

sex and longevity: the world's greatest health secret

1 Would it add another dimension to your enjoyment of sex if you knew that it was actually helping to increase your longevity? That might well be the case. The evidence, I admit, is a little tricky, but still very suggestive.

One study, for instance, showed that middle-age men having sex twice a week were 50 percent less likely to die prematurely than men enjoying sex less often.

A Duke University study that followed both men and women for 25 years found that, on average, the longevity of the men was directly and positively related to their frequency of sex, while in women the association was between longevity and their *enjoyment* of sexual relations.

The obvious problem with studies like these is that one could reasonably conclude that people with problems like poor circulation, high cholesterol, and high blood pressure have sex less often because of the sex-numbing effects of illness, rather than having worse health because of less sex. But wait...

A study conducted in Wales that statistically controlled for confounding factors like age and overall health *still* found a positive relationship between orgasm frequency and longevity.

Another study, carried out among college students, who are very unlikely to have chronic disease or impaired circulation, found that students having sex at least once a week had stronger immune systems than students having less sex. This suggests that sex may have an overall "tonic" effect, which could well translate into greater longevity.

In *For Women Only*, the doctors Jennifer and Laura Berman cite work by the University of Chicago's Michael Ruizen, M.D., a specialist in problems of senior citizens. In his book *Real Age: Are You as Young as You Can Be?* he calculates from various studies that having sex twice a week can add nearly 2 years to your life, while good sex every day can add 8!

If that's even close to the truth, sex might be the most underappreciated health practice going. I mean, when was the last time you saw a booklet in your doctor's office called "Just Do It"?

At least one doctor, Daniel Stein, M.D., of Tampa, calls sex a "significant public health concern" that deserves to take its place right up there along with exercise, a good diet, and vitamins.

So, you might not only add a new dimension of satisfaction to your sex life, knowing how good it is for you both, but also maybe even plan on having more sex in the bargain!

the world's shortest
sex tip

2

Chocolate Redi-Whip.

---

make your dreams
come true

3

"I had this dream last night, honey. A very vivid dream. You were (fill in with a sexual act of your choosing) and I was (fill in)."

"Oh? Was that exciting?"

"Incredibly. When I woke up, I was hard as a rock."

Now, if your lover has an IQ higher than her body temperature, she will realize that you aren't describing a literal dream, but a strong desire you are aching to have fulfilled. Still, it may be worth telling such a story.

Judith Scherven, Ph.D., says that women, even in today's world, are led to believe they should be "good girls." And, let's face it: sucking a peppermint while sucking a man's penis is not necessarily on her list of good-girl stuff. Dr. Scherven suggests describing your vision of her doing something wild, which gives her a needed sense of permission.

Are there men who need permission? My guess is yes; *lots*.

"Honey, I had this dream last night. It was about you—you and this amazing vibrator…"

---

sex
with satan

This may horrify and disgust you. But after trying it, your horror may develop shades of horny, and your disgust may morph into moan. What we have here is the Snake Charm-Her, a serpent-shaped vibrator, whose evil tail you can twist any which way you want him to tempt you. The multi-speed battery pack can make him slither or writhe. **Best of all:** Serpy's tongue flickers against your clit! Eve's revenge is available from *www.xandria.com*.

coitus interruptus heartburnus

5 Of all the causes of interrupted sex, some may be more embarrassing, but few are more painful than heartburn. Although they don't talk about it much on all those TV ads for heartburn medications, the fact is that heartburn can ruin sex, and sex can actually *cause* heartburn (also called gastro-esophageal reflux disorder or GERD).

What? Your doctor didn't tell you that getting laid can bring on an attack? Well, it can, and the key word here is "laid."

After eating a meal, if you lie down, the acidified contents of your stomach slosh up against the sphincter that separates your tummy from your esophagus. For most people, no harm is done; the sphincter stays shut. But for the millions of people who are prone to GERD, the acid-laden juices get through a sloppily closed sphincter and start burning the hell out of the tender esophagus.

If you're among those millions, you are vulnerable if your love tryst occurs shortly after a meal. Having somebody lying on your stomach doesn't help matters any!

To protect the sanctity of your sex, avoid lying down after eating a meal. Avoid large meals altogether near bedtime. If you crave sex at the wrong time, assume an upright position.

And there are certain foods known to help relax that already too-relaxed sphincter we mentioned: among them are coffee, alcohol, fat, chocolate, and mint. Strangely, every single one of these bad boys is in the after-dinner drink called Dutch coffee, the ingredients of which include Vandermint liqueur (alcohol, chocolate, and mint), coffee, and whipped cream (for the fat). That's one nightcap you should never, ever drink if you're prone to attacks of heartburn!

lover's quarrel
sex

Quarrels are inevitable between lovers. And we know, as mentioned before, that quarreling rouses testosterone and can make for especially great sex. Here is how the ancient Indian sex guide, *Kama Sutra*, describes a first-rate quarrel *cum* sex.

Something happens. And not that minor, either. Perhaps he accidentally calls her by another woman's name. "Then there is a great quarrel, with weeping, anguish, tossing hair, slaps, falling from the bed onto the ground, tearing off garlands and jewelry, and sleeping on the floor."

If we assume the man is at the bottom of the spat, he must throw himself at her feet, beg forgiveness, and coax, if not carry, her back into bed.

She lets herself be coaxed, but all the while she continues to goad him ("You drive me *crazy!*") and pulls at his hair or squeezes him so hard it hurts. She gives herself up to him, yet, even once he is inside her, and she's grinding against him, she doesn't stop the harping and hair pulling. **Result:** Lover's quarrel segues into emotionally wild sex!

the world's longest tease: **strip chess**

No, I'm serious! Consider first that people who play chess usually have a highly developed visual sense. And, if they happen to be male, their enjoyment of watching a female disrobe is matched by few other kicks (even including, in one survey, receiving oral sex). So strip chess is a natural.

Moreover, it is the only way on Earth you can literally undress someone using the power of your mind! So for horny intellectuals, we're talking nirvana.

It's best played when you have plenty of time and not much else to do, like a long rainy weekend day. Your table should be put in a warm part of the house, where you will not be visible to chess peeping toms. Snacks and drinks should be nearby, so you don't have to parade around in a state of partial undress.

Each player should wear no more than six items of clothing: shoes, socks, underpants, bra or undershirt, a top, and a bottom. Every time a player loses a game, he or she must remove one item of clothing. Jewelry, specs, lip rings, and the like do not count as clothing.

If a game ends in a stalemate, both players must remove a piece of clothing.

When one player is totally naked, the loser must then obey the winner's sexual wishes completely—how, where, and when.

If the slow pace of strip chess seems a bit daunting, you can shorten it in a couple ways. First, you can both start barefoot. That does away with four games right there. Second, you can play "speed chess," wherein each player has only 30 seconds to make a move. That adds an element of desperation that can only increase the erotic appeal of this noble, naughty game.

which variety
do you prefer?

"There is need for variety in sex but not in love."
—Theodore Reik

Reik was one of the most brilliant and readable of mid-20th-century shrinks. Unfortunately, it seems that lots of people twist his advice around, spicing up their lives with new love interests instead of new sexual adventures with the person they came to the dance with.

It is undeniable that a new "love" affair adds tremendous excitement to lovemaking. And some people need this excitement the way other people seem to need antidepressants.

Funny thing is, I'd wager that 90 percent of the time, these unfaithful partners are performing the very same kind of sexual acts with their new loves that they usually do at home. So, how long will it take for monotony to set back in? It's usually a matter of weeks, maybe months, not years.

Isn't it better to add variety to your sex, as Reik suggests, than go through all the heartache and mess that changing partners so often entails? Not that I'm suggesting that this book is some kind of "happy marriage" manual, but, well, yes I am!

massage her
to insanity

9 Set the stage for a long, sensual massage. There's soft music. An aromatic candle or two. Your supply of good massage oil, and maybe a towel. The recipient—let's say it's *she*—is butt naked. No modesty sheet, like they use in spas.

As she lies on her tummy, you begin by gently kneading her neck and shoulders—places that seem to hold more tension than any other in the human body. Slowly you work down her back. But when you get to her lovely butt, you *skip* it, just like a professional masseur would. Begin on the backs of her thighs and work down to her ankles, then her feet. When her feet have been softened to mush, have her turn over.

As you work your way down her front, being much gentler than you were on her back, you again pointedly skip her breasts and vaginal area. You get close—*real close*—but no touching.

When you reach the tops of her feet, go back to her erotic zones and get even closer than before. And as you get closer and closer, put your mouth right over those intimate areas and tell them how beautiful they are, and what you want to do to them.

When they tell you they *demand* to be massaged, too, whether with your hands or perhaps a vibrator, only then do you oblige.

Proceed in reverse order of sensitivity—butt first, then breasts, then vagina, then clitoris. If the man is the one receiving the massage, his rear-end should be kneaded very close to his anus, then his perineum (just below his testes), then the sack, and finally his penis.

Replenish massage oil often; many people find the sensation of oil on their skin adds another dimension of pleasure.

the chemistry
of love notes

10 Your lover *expects* a warm, affectionate note or card on Valentine's Day and her birthday. Though it's appreciated, it doesn't have the *surprise factor* we've talked about, that special zing to the feel-good brain center. Likewise, spoken words of affection are certainly appreciated, but they don't have that special added value of a written message. **Moral:** Give her a billet-doux when she doesn't expect it, and write it, preferably in longhand.

Just writing something like "You made me so happy last night. I'm the luckiest guy in the world!" is fine. If you write it on a romantic, quality sheet of paper, so much the better. But also try to do something unusual, *really* unexpected.

Create a "personal" want-ad in which you express a desire to find a lover who has very special qualities—*all of which your current lover has.* "Married redneck military man seeks woman, age 33, with interests in golf, bass fishing, quilting, and managing household budgets. Must look fabulous in denim shorts, have adorable breasts, skin like silk, and a smile that makes me melt. Purpose: love forever, and incredible sex. Applicants should meet me in bed at 11:00 P.M. for personal interview."

Tape the "ad" to the front page of her newspaper.

Fantasy #15
sex with joan of arc

For some puerile reason, I have always imagined Joan to be hot, and I mean before they burned her. Likewise, I'm sure many women have fantasized about having King Arthur or Richard the Lion-Hearted as a lover. That medieval look has a certain appeal, especially when you strip away some of that annoying heavy armor and get down to see some medieval skin.

Joan and Richard and their like can be re-created in your real-life fantasy with a wonderful see-through chain mail outfit. This is very classy, realistic looking, and soft enough to wear comfortably as you re-create the romance of yesteryear. There are several pieces, including a long shirt and a terrific headpiece. It's a unisex look, so you can be the saint or king. Available from *www.store.yahoo.com. sassyangel*.

gift for
a porny guy

12

This is a fun joke gift for the guy spending way too much time surfing the net or working on his laptop. You'll have to come up with any "legitimate" reasons to give him this offbeat (or beat-off) kit that masturbates him while he's on his computer. Talk about working on his "laptop!"

The Power Stroker is hooked up to the USB port of a computer, and features a lifelike masturbation sleeve that he can run through no less than ten speeds. It also has ten functions, including the ever-popular "Random," so he won't know what's coming next—unless it's him. (Available from *www.bettersex.com.*)

shock sex #8
bawdy body language

13

You're wearing something very sexy. But maybe he's getting used to it and isn't as instantly turned on as he was before. Try *this*.

Sit in front of him. Draw closer. He'll say, "What's that around your neck? What does it say?"

"Oh, you mean this choker? Read it."

He gets closer and reads: "*I   Cock.*"

Is that a little too strong a message? How about: "*I   Cum.*"

Not strong enough? Okay, there's always: "*F-ck Me.*"

These and many other messages (like "Bitch," "Slave," etc.) available from *www.wickedtemptations.com*.

water world **sex**

14 Enjoying sex surrounded by water adds a delicious new dimension to the experience. You can do it casually and impulsively, simply by jumping into the shower with your lover, or planning something special.

As warm water is filling the tub, light some scented candles and turn out the lights. The steam and the candlelight will create an extremely romantic fog. Pour lots of bubble bath into the tub and when there's a rich topping, you and she can slip in.

Face one another, if you like, and play footsie. Dr. Alex Comfort is a fan of big-toe sex—using the pad of the big toe to massage her clitoris—so if you want to, now's a good time to give it a go. Rub her feet, concentrating on the balls, but also rubbing the Achilles' tendon area, where there are supposedly connections to the center of sexual desire.

Change positions so you're sitting behind her, where you can soap up her body, massage her scalp, then reach around to fondle and stimulate her with your sudsy hands or a soft sponge (not a bath "puff"). Then she can sit behind you and give your penis a slow, rhythmic cleansing. (Any massaging of the neck and shoulders is a big bonus!)

You can then sit face-to-face with legs intertwined and have relations in the water, or slip out, wrap each other in big warm towels, and scurry off to bed.

For added fun, there are many waterproof sex toys. You might also want the Lover's Spa Kit from *www.affections.com*, which includes a soft, sensual sponge, a coconut water scoop, tropical bath oils, tea candles, and an "invitation card" to give to your partner. For a laugh, and more, look at the site's "anti-sagging balls cream" and "anti-sagging tits cream." Rub in well!

The *shower* is also a great venue for water-world sex. Avoid inserting a really soapy penis into a vagina, and use some extra lubrication. Also suggested: a thick, soft shower mat, so you won't slip... and you can protect your knees when it's your turn to go down.

---

sex on a
bearskin rug

15

Making love in front of a fireplace on a bearskin rug was the iconic sex scene in movies made a half-century ago. Want could be more delicious than rolling around naked with your sweetheart on luxurious fur?

How about luxurious faux fur? Real bearskins cost in the thousands of dollars, and may not be your cup of tea if you don't like the idea of turning Smokey into a mattress.

Luckily, we found marvelous faux bearskins at Cabela's, the fantastic hunting–fishing–outdoor-stuff store, at very reasonable prices (*www.cabelas.com*). A great Christmas present for both of you!

playing percussion
with his penis

16 For some strange reason, many men will respond more dramatically to this approach than they do to even the best tender licking and sucking. Actually, the two need to be used in tandem for best results.

While giving him oral sex, stop for a few seconds and "slap" his penis a time or two against your cheek. Or your tongue. Better, both. This will stiffen many guys instantly. Or, you can gently tap his erect penis with one hand against the palm of the other. Slapping it against your breasts is a real winner.

You can also use your hands for some percussive excitement on his drumstick. Use the tips of your fingers to tap very quickly up and down his penis and all around, like you were playing a saxophone.

the vibrating candy cane

17

A great little Christmas gift for the woman who has everything... except a foot-long red-and-white-striped vibrator in the shape of a candy cane. The smooth, rounded curved end should taste really sweet to her G-spot! (Available from *www.lingeriegifts.com*.)

the maiden's
divided mind
(and legs)

18

In your fantasy, he's forcing himself on you—that handsome brute—and like a good girl, you're trying to get him off you. At the same time, you're trying to get him off, period, and yourself as well. Here's the geometry to go along with your duplicitous passions.

You're on your back, with both your legs drawn forward. One thigh (of the "No" leg) is pressed against your breasts, and your foot is square on his chest, with which you rhythmically push him back—but not too far back. Your other leg (the "Yes" leg) is draped across his shoulder.

Result: You're stretched, creating even more pleasure for both of you as he thrusts deeply into your vault.

outrageous stocking
stuffers for her

19

(She's Been Naughty *and* Nice!) Here are a few things to put in her stocking, all compact and very inexpensive—$5 to $10 each.

Does she misplace her car keys all the time, but her vibrator, never? Here's the solution: the Micro Vibro Keychain, a small vibrator hooked to a keychain.

One of the cheapest thrills ever: a five-dollar pair of Nipple Suckers. A few squeezes and she's erect... and surprisingly excited. A must for photo shoots!

Another cheap thrill is the Clit Clip, an adjustable little thing with dangling black beads for a touch of style. (All of the above are available from *www.lingerietoys.inadult.com.*)

Give her a collection of 40 assorted Tasty Tattoos; tell her to lick 'em and stick 'em wherever she wants you to eat them off her. (Available from *www.lingeriexox.com.*)

Glitter and nudity go together like love and marriage, so give her a jar of Stardust Rainbow Body Glitter and she can adorn herself for your mutual admiration. (Available from *www.dear-lady.com.*)

Imagine entering a totally dark bedroom only to see a sex message mysteriously glowing on her naked body! That's what will be in store once she gets the Glow-in-the-Dark finger paint offered at *www.store1.yimg.com.*

3

conquering
hero

20

When the man wants to be in the position of a conqueror, she lies on her back, then raises not just her hips, but the small of her back off the bed. Her legs go way back, beyond her head, touching the headboard or wall. She cooperates with the conquest scenario by grasping her ankles to keep her legs well split and her feet far backward. The man must support himself on his hands, with his arms extended and placed just inside hers.

Hot and deeply penetrating: the sexual equivalent of Ben Gay!

---

outrageous stocking
stuffers for him

21

Here are a few compact and inexpensive holiday gifts—cheap and tawdry, like your guy.

First something that's actually very sweet: Tantric Foot Massage Cream, full of mysterious and erotic herbs and oils that will bliss him out when you rub it into his hooves. (Available from *www.ShopInPrivate.com*.)

Every real man needs a cock ring, and the Adjustable Loop Enhancer is not only the cheapest I've seen, but unlike most, is fully and quickly adjustable. (Available from *www.shop.sex-superstore.com*.)

Tired of sucking Altoids? Heat up his oral sex with Good Head Oral Delight Gel (Mystical Mint), available from *www.dear-lady.com.*

Here's a way to give him oral sex without getting neck strain. The Oro-Simulator consists of a short latex sleeve that fits over the top of his penis, and is connected to a hand-held pump. First, you lube his tube, then slip on the sleeve and pump away, giving him a sensation said to be a lot like oral sex (*www.stockroom.com*).

have a talent show
between your legs

22

TV "reality shows" have a certain fascination, but one thing I don't like about them is their overwhelming negativity. It's always, "The tribe has spoken; get the hell off the island!" or "I said, 'You're *fired!*' not 'You're *hired*,' you moron!"

This is a kind of *entirely positive* reality show that takes place between your legs (and possibly elsewhere), and involves his various tongue and hand moves competing with one another to see which ones get the top prizes from you, the sole judge. The purpose is not just to get him to do 50 different things to you (well, that too), but to give him permission to try everything he can come up with—without appearing to be a totally confused novice with attention deficit disorder.

Here's how it works. If what he's doing feels really good, say, "That's good." If it doesn't feel that good, don't say *anything* negative ("What are you *doing* down there?"); just say, "Okay." That means it's time for him to move on. Until he hears your "Okay" he keeps at it, for better or worse.

Now, you may not be able tell exactly what he's doing in any particular act, so he'll have to try to remember what he was doing when you said, "That's good." You can help him remember the really good moves by saying, "Remember that!"

With honest work, he should be able to do at least a few dozen things in his me-vs.-me talent show. When he has exhausted his current repertoire, it's time for the semi-finals, where he does encores of the potential winners. Finally, you announce the Third Place, Second Place, and First Place champions. When you're good and ready, give some kind of reward for all his hard work.

Some of the moves he can put on the stage might include the Battle of the Clitoral Bands, where he progresses from tongue flicks to tongue licks to kissing... sucking... using his nose... changing direction... involving two fingers, three, four... even tapping it or gently twisting it like it's a toothpaste tube cap. He can stretch your lips apart for better access, massage your mound of Venus, and rub his chin at the base of your vagina.

You can assist his talent show by asking him to move to a different position or by moving your own body. How does it feel when he's by your side versus between your legs? You sitting over his face, toward him, versus facing his feet? One leg draped around him, or two? Worth trying: kneel, face the headboard of the bed, lean on it, spread your legs, and have him lie under you, and give you oral sex, while one of his hands fondles a breast and the other massages your perineum, just under the vagina.

There's no rule in the game that says he can't have an assistant joining the talent show: a vibrator, for instance.

sexy
santa outfits

23 Last Christmas Eve, for the first time ever, my wife stunned me by waltzing down the stairs in a very erotic Santa outfit, from a furry red cap to sexy black stockings. In between, a saucy bustier with garters and a thong. I eventually recovered and we had a very special, intimate holiday evening in front of the fireplace.

A site with lots of appealing Santa outfits is *www.flirtylingerie. com*. One, called Santa's Mistress, is especially nice: sexy (with a long bare midriff) but not over the top. Getting closer to the top is a three-piece outfit consisting of a cute fake fur hat, bra, garter belt, and G-string set. Make sure your house is warm before putting this one on!

If you *do* want to go over the top, there's the Santa's Girl Boobs Out Baby Doll outfit. Sing "Have Yourself a Merry Little Christmas" as you come downstairs in this number!

Yes, there are Santa outfits for guys, though they're not as elaborate or fetching as the ones for women. Have a look at something like the Sexy Santa, with satin boxers, a shiny black belt, elastic suspenders to go over your bare chest, and a Santa hat, at *www.lingeriegifts.com*. If you want a minimalist outfit, try their velvet G-string, featuring a white beard.

christmas eve
sex

24 One of you is tired, maybe both. But as you lie there in your bed (finally!), visions of sugarplums come into his head, and candy canes into hers. For an easy, intimate connection, try this.

She is lying on her back. Her man is next to her, but on his side. It's best if he's on his left side if he's a righty. She then lifts her right leg, and the man slips his right leg between both of hers. She then wraps her other leg around him, enveloping him. He enters her sidewise.

A physician specializing in such matters says this position is not only easy, because both partners are lying down, but has the bonus of the man's topmost leg applying some extra pressure to the woman's clitoris. It's all very intimate, too.

heal a cut
with sex

The term *sexual healing* is usually used to mean that loving sex can help heal the wounded mind or spirit. But unbeknownst to most people is that good sex can heal a physical injury, too.

Researchers at Ohio State University gave volunteers minor boo-boos on their skin, then watched carefully for a few days to see how quickly they healed. They found that the people who had the lowest levels of cortisol—the notorious stress hormone—healed fastest. And who had the lowest levels of this killer hormone? Those with the happiest marriages, the researchers found.

Since frequent, satisfying sex is an important determinant of happy marriages, it seems to me that sex can therefore be said to—okay, indirectly—heal physical injuries. Take your boo-boo to bed with your lover and both of you may come out the happier.